FEELING
& HEALING
YOUR
EMOTIONS

Conrad W. Baars, M.D.

Logos International
Plainfield, New Jersey

Dedicated
to
all Christians

FEELING AND HEALING YOUR EMOTIONS
Copyright © 1979 by Logos International
All rights reserved
Printed in the United States of America
Library of Congress Catalog Card Number: 79-53629
International Standard Book Number: 0-88270-384-6
Logos International, Plainfield, New Jersey 07060

Table of Contents

Chapter 1

The Feeling Revolution

"It is the *feeling* of the President of the United States that the price of imported oil is too high."

"The psychiatrists and psychologists on the panel were almost unanimous in their *feeling* that masturbation is quite natural and normal."

"FDA researchers cannot help but *feel* that Laetrile is useless in the treatment of cancer."

"Several leading economists were asked for their *feelings* about the reason for the sudden drop in the stock market."

"The newly appointed advisor to the president stated in a press conference that she has the strong *feeling* that abortion is a matter of choice for the woman."

"Several theologians wrote a book on the subject of human sexuality because they *felt* that the moral standards of the Church cause unnecessary hardships for the average Catholic."

The psychiatrist-author of a learned book about feelings writes: "I have never *felt* that people's inner feelings have some claim to public recognition. . . . I myself *feel* we have responsibility to keep 'it' (bad temper, foul language, ill humor) in."

These are but a very few examples of how we have become a nation of "feelers." Or, at least, if we still think, know, believe, and have opinions, we do not care to say so. We prefer to call it "feeling." Check your newspapers and magazines and you will discover that "to feel that" is used frequently to express activity of our reasoning faculty. Listen to relatives, friends, neighbors, fellow workers, hosts and guests of TV talk shows, and you will hear them do the same thing.

There is no doubt about it—feeling is IN! But is thinking on the way out? Is man's reason becoming an endangered species?

"If it feels good, do it!" many a bumper sticker proclaims.

We are told: "Let it all hang out. Do your own thing. Follow your feelings. Express your emotions. Never repress your feelings."

You are O.K. and I am O.K. and everybody is O.K.! And everything you do with another person is O.K., as long as you *really love* him. But what is "really"? And what is "love"? A feeling pure and simple? Or something more than feeling?

We have come a long way from Victorian prudery, unemotional formality and stiff upper lips, to our present day enthusiasm for feeling, hugging, kissing and touching everyone we meet. Those of us who drag our feet in participating in this feeling revolution are gently asked on bumper stickers whether we have hugged our kids today.

Sex, of course, has provided the most fertile soil for the feeling revolution. The new feeling philosophy has developed into a veritable sexual arena of novel experimentations, unrestrained gratifications, fanciful titillations, unpurged audiovisual presentations and publications, and new anything-goes legislation.

The last stronghold of "emotional uptightness"—angry feelings—is being attacked with great vigor by an army of self-acclaimed assertiveness experts. People are trained by them to express their anger and to "tell it like it is." They learn new ways of "looking out for number one," and to "go with their anger." No one is allowed to be shy, meek or self-effacing any more.

You ask, how do *I* feel about this feeling revolution? If you really mean what you say, "How do I *feel*," the answer is, "Both glad and sad." If you mean, however, "What do I *think*?", I will give you my professional opinion. First, I will give you the good news—the reason for my feeling glad.

Much good has come from Sigmund Freud's discovery early in this century to the effect that the neurotic repression of our emotions and feelings is detrimental to our emotional health. The once high incidence of sexual neuroses has dwindled to almost zero, although not all older persons have been able to shake off the effects of the damage done in their childhood years.

We have learned how important it is to make our children *feel* loved by showing affection. Bottle feeding is making way of late for old-time breast feeding as parent-infant bonding—the intimate relationship of infants to their mothers that may be formed immediately after birth—is sought in skin-to-skin and eye-to-eye contact. Birthing centers are being established in some hospitals for fear that, unless we get back into the family business, the country is on a headlong course for disaster in terms of human relationships and family interactions.

In general people are becoming freer and more spontaneous in relating to others also on a feeling level. They want to learn more about emotions and feelings, and how they can contribute to a more contented and happier existence. Their instinctive substitution of "feeling" for "thinking" is an indication of their awareness that in the past we have stressed the development of our thinking mind at the expense of the use of our emotions. By saying "I feel" instead of "I think," people mean, "We want things to change; we want to be *whole* human beings, not solely thinking human beings."

Much progress has been made in controlling or lessening unpleasant feelings like anxiety, depression, despair, agitation and tension with a large variety of tranquilizers and antidepressant medication. Many physical disorders can now be treated successfully because of what we have learned about the relationship between body and feelings. Nevertheless, we still have a long way to go before our understanding of emotions and our treatment of emotional disorders can be considered adequate and successful.

Now for the bad news—the reason for my feeling sad.
Our failure to substitute for past neurotic repression of
feelings and emotions a non-neurotic manner of dealing
with them is having wide repercussions throughout our
society. This is most evident in the sexual area, the prime
target of the popular belief that to exercise restraint is a
certain invitation to become neurotic, or stay emotionally
retarded and unfulfilled.

Instead of sexual neuroses we now see other sexual
dysfunctions and new forms of emotional immaturity.
With all its pleasures, the so-called sexual revolution is
producing more impotent playboys and frigid playmates.[1]
With the greatly increased "sexual freedom" there is
more post-coital depression and greater inability to relate
in non-genital ways. These sexually, or rather genitally,
hyperactive persons are more lonely and isolated from
each other. They frustrate each other in their
promiscuous pursuit of the goal: to feel loved and wanted.
The "joys of sex" are accompanied by intensified feelings
of fear, worry, anxiety, tension, hate, loneliness,
depression and despair.

Ignorance about how to deal maturely with our sexual
feelings, together with continued suppression and
repression of our so-called "negative" emotions—especially anger in all its variations and
nuances—as well as generalized confusion about the role
of emotions and feelings in our lives, are responsible for
the me-first culture of self-fulfilment and the new
narcissism, "the besetting psychological disorder of
modern western culture."[2]
The speculations about this modern disorder by

psychoanalysts, psychiatrists, sociologists, social historians, social critics and psychologists reveal the extent of our inability to put man's emotions and feelings in their proper context. The conclusions of these human scientists, varied as they are, make it abundantly clear that modern man is not served by our continuing need to see the individual as a social animal, or a rational animal, or a behavior phenomenon. Man is *not* an animal, even though he feels pain and pleasure like an animal. He is *not* a rock even though he falls like a rock. Men and women are rock-like, plant-like, animal-like, and God-like; but they are not rocks, plants, animals, or gods. They are entirely just human beings, human persons.[3]

Man must be seen and understood as man, as the sum total of all his faculties—*vegetative* (pertaining to the plant functions of nutrition, growth and reproduction), *sensory* (pertaining to the animal functions of sensing, feeling and moving), *intellectual*, *volitional* (pertaining to the will), and *spiritual* in his relationship to his fellow-man and his Creator. Only in this context is it possible to make sense of what always has been, in a certain way, the most puzzling aspect of his nature: his emotional life.

Therefore, a book that intends to shed light on the precise purpose and function of man's emotions and feelings must give due consideration to the spiritual dimension of man. To exclude this dimension, as most books on psychology and psychiatry do, is, in my opinion, unscientific, regardless of the more widely held belief that scientific study must be limited to the scientifically measurable.

The reader will have to determine for himself who or what is true in this regard. For sure, many a reader may no longer know whether what he experiences is a matter of feeling or knowing. As a result he may be confused about many issues of vital importance to his state of life. His inability to extricate himself from this confusion is often a cause of apathy (from the Latin, *apathos*, "without feeling or passion"). Without clarity of thinking and a fully developed and balanced emotional life, he is defenseless against the powers of evil. He is weak.

However, as he gains insight into the differences between feeling and thinking, and into the ways each can support and strengthen the other, his powers of judgment will multiply. So will his capacity for knowing and living the good news, for leading the life Jesus wants him to have in abundance.

For those afflicted by emotional disorders this insight will help lift their confusion so they can benefit more from psychotherapy. Those in positions of influence and power over others will be better disposed to make correct judgments unaffected by undue emotional contamination. Their greater love and compassion for their children, students, employees, religious subjects, constituents, and others, will make their laws and regulations more humane without abandonment of basic principles of morality, justice and charity.

This book is dedicated to all Christians. My reason for doing so is twofold. First, because through the centuries too many Christians of all denominations have been the unfortunate victims of emotional—and indirectly, spiritual—afflictions which in some way are traceable to misconceptions of emotions in the Christian culture and to misunderstandings of certain Scripture passages.

Second, because I am grateful for all I have learned from my Christian patients, as well as my Christian audiences and correspondents throughout North America and other parts of the world.

In dedicating this book to all Catholics, Protestants, and Evangelicals it is my sincere wish that it will contribute to greater unity among my Christian brothers and sisters, and bring to them and the world the peace and joy of Christ through the healing and prevention of emotional suffering.

When I write about the meaning of man's emotional life as an integral, well-defined part of his God-given nature, I do so as a Christian psychiatrist, not as a humanist. I am convinced that even those who have been taught that psychology and psychiatry are of the devil, those who believe these sciences belong to the "world," will agree that I am not a secular humanist, but a true Christian after reading this book. I am equally convinced that this book will deepen the reader's belief in the healing power of the Holy Spirit, as well as his understanding of how the Spirit works with and through human beings. He may be assured that the contents of these pages will not lead him away from the gospel, or ensnare him in strictly human ways of thinking.

This book is written in question-and-answer style with a minimum of professional jargon. Whenever their use could not be avoided, professional terms are explained and clarified.

It is written primarily for nonprofessionals, ordinary men and women who form the backbone of our society, as well as people in positions of leadership in business, churches, government, the military, and elsewhere. It is intended for parents and teachers, adults and adolescents, laity and religious. In short, it is for everyone who desires to enrich his or her life by learning the exact meaning and interdependency of emotions and feelings, feeling and thinking, heart and mind, being and doing, restraint and repression, the flesh and the spirit, soma and psyche.

NOTE: This is not to say that professionals, psychiatrists, psychologists, psychotherapists, counselors, theologians, pastoral workers, spiritual directors, and all workers in the mental health field cannot benefit from this book. They can. In fact, *Feeling and Healing Your Emotions* is a suitable introduction to those books—the ones I've already written or co-authored and others I plan to write—designed for the professional reader.[4]

Chapter 2

Emotions–Man's Psychic Motors

Q. Dr. Baars, I am confused about the words "emotions" and "feelings." Are they the same?

A. Not quite. Though one can say that all emotions are feelings, the reverse in not true. Not all feelings are emotions.

Feelings that are not emotions include, for example, those of pain, hunger, thirst, cold, warmth, fatigue, tension, relaxation, sleepiness, and dizziness. These feelings originate in our body and cause us to be aware of certain changes in a part or the whole of our body, or any of its organs. These somatic feelings, or bodily sensations, serve the purpose of alerting us to our bodily conditions and needs, and of giving us an opportunity to make adjustments to bring about or maintain a healthy or comfortable bodily state. For example, we eat in response to the feeling of hunger; we take a rest when we feel tired;

we go for a checkup when we feel pain; we turn on the heat when we feel cold.

An emotion, on the other hand, is primarily a psychic reaction to stimuli from the world around us. As we are part of that world, too, we can also feel an emotion in response to our own thoughts, memories and bodily feelings. It is a response to whatever information our senses provide concerning the goodness, lack of goodness, usefulness or harmfulness things and beings have for us.

For example, I love a gorgeous sunset; I desire to buy a beautiful painting; I feel joy when I am with my children; I hate burned food; I feel aversion whenever I must take my foul-tasting medicine; I feel sad when I am sick; I hope to pass my exam; I despair of ever making enough money to buy a house; though I fear a fist fight your words give me courage to defend myself; getting bad advice from my broker makes me angry. I will come back later to a discussion of these eleven basic human emotions. Right now I want to draw your attention to the meaning of the word "emotion."

Derived from the Latin, *ex-motus*, past participle of the verb *ex-movēre*, the word "emotion" has to do with *motion, movement, motor*. Emotions, like the bodily or somatic feelings, cause us "to be moved" or "move," depending on the particular kind of information our senses give us. But unlike the feelings which are concerned mainly with the state of our body and its organs, our emotions are reactions to the world around us and to our own inner psychic world. In that sense one can say that their importance overshadows that of our bodily feelings because their range is infinitely great. On the other hand, if we were not enabled by our somatic feelings to take good care of our bodies we would not be around very long to be moved emotionally by the world we live in.

Bodily feelings are easily understood and dealt with by all of us. Our emotions are much more complex and therefore a ready source of confusion and misdirection. Our current "feeling revolution" primarily involves our emotions, not our somatic feelings.

Q. That means our sexual feelings, in which we see the greatest upheaval and lack of inhibition and control, belong to the emotions. Is that right?

A. Not really. Sexual feelings result from the stimulation of specific end organs in our erogenous zones, in the same manner that pain is felt when specific end organs in the skin, bones, internal organs, and so forth are stimulated. Once these sexual feelings have been experienced by self-stimulation, arousal by others, or watching things of a sexual nature, they may then be felt when we think of the person we love intimately, or by any other thoughts, fantasies, and memories with sexual connotations.

However, just because sexual feelings can originate in the thinking mind or be closely associated with the emotion of love, does not mean they are emotions. We all know that the smell of fresh bread baking in the oven can make us "hungry," or rather evoke a hearty appetite. So can the thought of going to the best restaurant in town in a few hours. When I was imprisoned in France during World War II some of the French prisoners would spend hours recounting in detail every imaginable culinary delight. This would intensify my hunger pains to the point of having to request them to change the subject. Likewise, the very thought, when we wake up, of the backbreaking work to be done that day can make us feel exhausted even before we start.

It is because our sexual feelings can be aroused so easily, and their pleasurable character can be so intense, that they have been in the forefront of our so-called "feeling revolution." And because they can be associated so very closely with our emotion of love we have been led to believe that the sexual revolution was a sign of greater emotional maturity.

I expect to make clear that this is an illusion. I also want to deal with what emotional maturity really entails, and everything else about your emotions you should have learned when you were a child and adolescent, but nobody ever told you.

Q. I like the idea of calling emotions "motors that cause movement." Are there different kinds of movement?

A. Yes, indeed. The easiest way to understand the different kinds of movement or functions which emotions can cause or have is by distinguishing two kinds of emotions or "motors."

One group of emotions causes inner movement within the psyche. This inner movement may be compared to that occurring in a light bulb when you flip the switch on. Electrons begin to move which create light and warmth. Thus it is also with the first group of emotions. We feel moved with *love* for our dearest friend. We are moved with *compassion* in seeing him sick in bed. His suffering makes us feel *sad* and moves us to tears. When he recovers we are moved with *joy*.

The second kind of movement is comparable to that of an electric motor. When the key is turned the motor begins to run and provides the source of energy for a car, an electric drill, a mechanical toy, and the like. Likewise, the emotions of this type provide the energy for our actions and deeds. More about this type of psychic motor later on.

First, I want to deal with the emotions which cause inner movement within the psyche, the emotions of the pleasure appetite. They function in their simplest and purest form in the child in response to the sense objects he can touch, see, hear, taste and smell. As he grows older and his intellectual and spiritual lives develop, he sees and evaluates the sense objects of his world in a changing light. They acquire higher or "nobler" qualities than the simple material qualities they possess in and by themselves. As a result the intellect increasingly modifies and "ennobles" the child's earliest emotional responses.

When we recognize something as being good and pleasurable for us, that sense object will stimulate in us the first and fundamental emotion of the pleasure appetite, namely the emotion of love. This feeling may grow into the emotion of desire, and when we come to possess that sense object we will experience the emotion of joy. To give an example, you "fall in love" with a beautiful dress; the longer you admire it in the window the stronger your desire to wear it becomes; finally, when you can afford to buy it, or someone presents it to you as a gift, you feel joyful.

The corresponding emotions for that which does not constitute a sense-good or an object of pleasure for us, in fact just the opposite—a sense-evil (here the word "evil" has nothing to do with morality; we are discussing only what is transpiring on the level of the senses)—are those of hate, aversion and sadness. When the doctor tells me I must take cod-liver oil for my anemia, I feel hate—"dislike," if you prefer—for this medicine; as I open the bottle when the moment arrives for me to take it, I feel aversion, or revulsion; and when I swallow it I feel anything but joy; I feel sad.

These six emotions make up the first group: love, desire and joy in response to whatever my senses recognize as a sense-good; hate, aversion and sadness in response to a sense-evil. Our language offers us a number of words to describe these basic emotions and their varied nuances, modifications, intensities and degrees. *Roget's Thesaurus* gives a selection of many words for all our emotions. Common variants for the emotion of love are *liking, fondness;* for desire—*wish, want;* for joy—*happiness, delight, gladness, pleasure, satisfaction,* and so on. For the emotion of hate it offers *dislike, displeasure, distaste;* for aversion—*repugnance, repulsion, disgust, loathing;* for sadness—*unhappiness, joylessness, sorrow, blues.*

There are also words that describe combinations of any of the emotions belonging to this group. *Compassion* connotes love and sadness; *tenderness,* love and gentleness, and so on. Sympathy, empathy, affection, kindness and a host of other words describe either combinations of several emotions, or nuances of a single emotion.

All of the emotions in this first group are called emotions of the "pleasure appetite," the inner movements of human beings aroused by all that is good, loveable and pleasurable. Because these emotions—when fully developed and integrated with our higher faculties—make us typically human, I like to call them "humane emotions." They make up the "heart" or inner core of man's emotional life.

Q. Are you suggesting that animals do not have the same or similar emotions because you call them "humane"? Are we not rational animals and therefore like them in everything except our rational faculty?

A. Although animals, at least the higher species, possess essentially the same emotions as humans, it is precisely because they lack a rational faculty that their emotions are not "ennobled." Let me explain. Emotions, in and by themselves, exist for the benefit of the one who possesses them. In this sense they can be said to be selfish; they serve their owner, first and foremost. Only under the growing influence of the intellect, which provides man with much more information about the world than the primary sources of our emotions—the senses—can ever give us, the emotions become oriented also toward the good of others.

A child feels joy when he possesses a beautiful toy; it is *his* toy. He is not happy when another child has a toy that he himself does not have. On the other hand, a mature adult may experience greater joy when not he but someone else possesses something valuable. The other's joy is also his joy. The child's *selfish* love, desire and joy become over the years the *selfless* love, desire, and joy of the mature adult. Animals do not love in this human way, even if at times they seem to behave as if they do.

Q. I have to give that some more thought. In the meantime, will you tell us about this second group of emotions you said we have?

A. As I said before, this group of emotions provide the energy for our actions. They stimulate us to move, to act, whether it is by talking, walking, writing, laboring, studying, or other activities. These actions are aimed at doing what is useful for the gratification of our desire to obtain something that will give us joy. Working at a menial job to earn money would be a very common example of a utilitarian activity that will enable us to buy something that will make us happy. Submitting to an operation so that one will enjoy good health is another one.

A moment's reflection will make it clear why we need a separate set of emotions to engage in some utilitarian activity. None of the humane emotions I have explained before will stimulate us to do whatever is useful, or difficult, or requires backbreaking labor, or whatever else needs to be done to overcome an obstacle that prevents us from enjoying something, or to protect ourselves from something harmful—cancer, for example—that keeps us from enjoying life. Most people enjoy having white, sparkling teeth and a perfect bite. But none love, desire or enjoy the hours of dental work or surgery it may require. A retired person finds delight in growing his own fruit and vegetables, yet he finds nothing desirable or enjoyable in constant weeding. It is clear that in either example the person needs some different kind of emotion to move him to exert effort.

The two basic emotions which may become operative when faced with the need to do something that is not enjoyable or desirable in itself, because it takes pain and effort, are (1) hope—or any of its variants, like confidence, trust, expectation, optimism; and (2) despair or hopelessness and pessimism. If we must prepare for a very difficult examination in order to obtain a desired diploma or license, we can react emotionally to this challenge either in an optimistic way with the emotion of hope and confidence; or pessimistically with a feeling of despair.

Our ultimate decision—to study or not to study for weeks and months on end without a rest or time for fun—will be greatly influenced, if not determined, by either of these two emotional responses. However, in a mature and healthy person the last word will be spoken by our higher faculty of the will, about which you will read more later.

There are still other emotions that also belong to this group, that which we have called the "utilitarian emotions." These serve the purpose of stimulating us to respond to whatever is harmful, to what threatens our life, safety, freedom, health, peace of mind, our loved ones, our possessions and so on. Again there are two ways of responding to a threat, namely either in an optimistic manner with the emotion of courage—boldness, fearlessness, fortitude, audacity, nerve, and the like; or pessimistically with the emotion of fear—or dread, timidity, fright, anxiety, or panic. Again, how we will actually act in the face of a danger or possible harm will be determined in the first instance by either of these two basic utilitarian emotions. But, unless there are pathologically chronic or momentary obstructions to the normal emotion-will relationship, the final action will be determined by the will.

Lastly, there is a fifth utilitarian emotion. It is, so to speak, the "ultimate emotion" that serves the purpose of emotionally arousing us when an evil is certain to harm us, or when it has already done so. For instance, my feeling of anger is aroused when somebody strikes me in the face—or you feel angry when you hear about plans to fire you from your job for no good reason. The anger is our ultimate stimulus to try and protect ourselves from almost certain harm; to try to undo the harm already done; to take measures that the harm is not done again in the future; to deal as effectively as possible with the cause of our feeling of anger. There are numerous synonyms and variants of the emotion of anger. To mention a few: irritation, annoyance, upset, hurt, mad, temper, wrath, resentment, ire.

These five basic emotions of the utility appetite therefore are very useful and necessary psychic motors in giving us the energy to overcome obstacles that separate us from the things we desire and which promise to make us joyful. They are also needed to arouse us in defense against what is harmful in the hope that, when successful, we will be happy. Of course, when despair or fear is the cause of our inaction, we will not succeed in overcoming the obstacle or protecting ourselves from harm, and thus we will be unhappy. Or, in other words, the humane emotions are responsible for our feelings of joy and happiness, while the utilitarian emotions operate in the service of the humane emotions by paving the way. The utilitarian emotions serve the humane emotions.

Q. I notice that love, desire, joy, hope, and courage have opposing emotions of hate, aversion, sadness, despair, and fear. What is the opposing emotion to anger?

A. There is none. Even if one is inclined to consider, as some do, the emotion of anger as a combination of the emotions of hate and courage—hate for the cancer that threatens life, and courage to fight it by every means possible—it would not follow that its opposite would be a combination of love and fear. There simply is none. Nevertheless, I would suggest that you give this question some thought. It will deepen your understanding of the emotions in general.

Q. If it is the true that our humane emotions are stimulated by what we know or sense is good for us (or not good), and our utilitarian emotions by what is useful or harmful, what organs or faculties provide us with this information?

A. The sense of knowledge of what is good for us, or pleasing to our nature, comes primarily from our external senses—sight, hearing, touch, taste and smell—as well as from our internal sense of imagination—by means of which we are able to imagine or visualize in our mind what is actually absent in our immediate environment. These senses directly stimulate our humane emotions. I feel happy when listening to my favorite music. When my wife calls me long distance I wish I could be with her. I feel happy when I know I have been promoted in my job, because I visualize or imagine what I can buy with the larger paycheck.

In this last example, we see how an abstract idea stimulates my humane emotions by means of the imagination. Take such an abstract idea as "freedom." When we try to form an idea of what it means we use images like prison gates opening or going away to college for the first time and not having your parents sit up waiting for you when you come home. Thoughts, ideas, opinions stimulate emotional responses via the products of the imagination.

It is somewhat less simple in the case of the utilitarian emotions. Animals know instinctively what is useful and harmful for them. For instance, a spider "knows" how to spin his web, and how to repair it when it is destroyed; a bird "knows" how to build its nest; the salmon "knows" where to go to spawn, and so on. But man's instinct is poorly developed. The infant's "knowledge" of how to nurse at its mother's breast seems to be the most developed one.

Perhaps in ages past man, too, possessed a much greater instinctive knowledge of what was useful and harmful to him. If so, one could speculate that it had less and less chance to develop in children because of their parents' eagerness to prematurely make them do useful things (roots of the work ethic), and warn them against potentially harmful things (roots of over-protectiveness). As a result of the parents' anxious need to protect their children and make them into achievers, children are prevented from discovering harmful and useful qualities naturally. Instead of relying on their own instincts they have been trained to rely on the "wisdom" of adults.

The word "sophisticated" is defined as: "1. altered by education, worldly experience; changed from the natural character or simplicity; artificial; 2. deceptive, misleading." Because of this, one could say that man possesses a "sophisticated instinct" because its natural character has been altered, evidently more for the bad than for the good. He has lost what perhaps once was a natural faculty. Since the child's natural instinct is practically nonexisting, and his education or training by adults or his worldly experience may be deceptive or misleading, it is precisely here that emotional malfunctions have a chance of developing. (See Chapter 6.)

To return to the question, what faculties stimulate our utilitarian emotions? It is this sophisticated instinct (or "particular reason" in rational psychology) as well as our memory that are the prime stimulators of our utilitarian psychic motors. Or, to narrow down the latter, it is our memory or recall of what we felt, and how we responded, and how these responses worked out earlier in life when faced with a variety of obstacles and dangers, that has an important bearing on how we respond emotionally as adults.

Q. Earlier you spoke of the ennobling effect of reason on our humane emotions. You also spoke of man's will. Can you tell us more about those higher faculties of reason and will?

A. On this higher level man—not the animal—possesses a third motor, a super-motor so to speak, which is, or should be, in charge of all our actions. It should have the final word in making decisions as to what actions one will take when we are moved by our emotions. Our super-motor, or free will, should make these decisions with the help of the information provided by our intellect (which in turn gets much of its information from the same senses which also stimulate the emotions). It should make its decisions in freedom, that is, unhampered by obstacles from without or from within (more about this later). If this super-motor operates in gear with, and supported by, the utilitarian emotions we will act smoothly, if not effortlessly.

For example, if we will to succeed in our studies at all cost and also feel hopeful about our ability to do so, our will is supported by our emotion of hope and things promise to go well. Our will is made truly powerful because of its support by hope. We have "will power." On the other hand, this power will be much less if, instead of hope, we feel inclined to despair. Now our will must work against this feeling of despair. Because the will's energy is diverted it is less powerful. The studies will go harder, though success is still possible, of course.

If our third psychic motor, our free will, is in gear with

our humane emotions we will act in a *truly human way*. For instance, if we share our riches with the poor because Jesus told us so, and we do it also because we are filled with compassion for them, our acts of charity have a truly human quality. This is not so, or much less so, when we will to be charitable but feel devoid of compassion for the poor. (Of course, this does not diminish the moral value of the charitable act. More on the role of our emotions in acts of virtue in a later chapter.)

Q. **You mean this free will, which you call our psychic super-motor, has the final say in how we act and feel? Or should have the final word?**
A. You are right as far as our actions are concerned. The will always has the final say as far as acting and doing are concerned. At least, this is true for the truly mature adult, who is free of emotional or mental illness, or organic brain disease, or any other abnormal condition that prevents the will from exercising its proper function without interference.

But the will cannot dictate or determine what we feel or should feel. Our psychic motors, our emotions, are stimulated by what we sense, imagine, know, or believe is good, bad, useful or harmful for us. The will, being also a psychic motor, is not a stimulant of our emotions. It cannot command how we are to feel, nor can *my* will command *your* emotions. Not even God can command us what to feel. But He can and does command how we are to act, and it is up to our free will to decide what course of action to take when we are emotionally aroused, and how to control and direct these acts.

In this regard we are also different from the animals, whose actions are determined by feelings. If there are several feelings at the same time, the strongest one determines the animal's actions. The animal has no higher faculty, neither free will, nor reason. We say that certain animals are "smart" but this smartness is not on a par with that of man who, for instance, knows what a tree is regardless of the great variety of existing trees. An animal "knows" only this tree, or that tree. He knows the tree with his senses because it looks and smells in a certain way. Man knows the universal tree as well as the particular tree; the animal "knows" only the particular tree.

The animal's feelings, aroused as they are by his senses, as well as by his instincts, determine how he will act. Unless he is trained to go against those feelings or instincts by a human being who conditions his responses with other feelings (fear of punishment or desire for reward), the animal acts on impulse. The animal acts more or less spontaneously according to what he feels. To act on impulse is natural for the animal, but not for man. His feelings and impulses to act require reflection by his intellect. When he is fully integrated on all levels of his nature, and possesses a well-directed will, he is able to act spontaneously and correctly! The animal, child and sociopath act more or less impulsively unless trained to do otherwise.

Q. If I have it right, our utilitarian emotions are motors for action, and so is our free will. Right?

A. Yes, you are quite correct. And that explains why there is, for example, confusion about the meaning of "maturity." Because our will can bring about any action that any of the five basic utilitarian emotions—singly or in combination—can move us to perform, it is possible for a person to live and act almost exclusively on his rational/volitional level (i.e., on his thinking/willing level), without being emotionally involved.

To give a simple example, when I catch somebody in the act of stealing my wallet my feeling of anger is capable of making my fist hit him (with or without consent of my will). But I can also hit that person without first feeling anger (either because I never allow myself to feel this emotion, or because I don't care since I know the wallet is empty). In that case I might *will* to hit him because I *think* he needs to be taught a lesson, or it is the best way to make him give me back my belonging. In the absence of any emotion my will decides how I will act.

As I shall illustrate later many people act almost all the time without participation of their emotions. What I want to point out here is that such a "cool and collected" way of life may easily give the impression of mature living. But it is not. A truly mature existence demands a harmonious integration between emotions, thinking and willing. Only then can we experience to the fullest the joy for which we are created. It is the absolute psychological foundation for the abundant life Jesus has brought us.

Q. What about the other part of our higher faculties, man's intellect?

A. Man derives his knowledge of the world first from his senses. This sense knowledge is of a concrete or particular nature and provides the material for our reason to work on, to analyze, synthesize, judge, abstract and so on. This source of higher knowledge is our reason, our working mind or discursive mind. Our reason enables us to reason, to argue, to think, form ideas, to compare, judge, solve problems. If we do all these things in a reasonable manner we are proceeding in a rational manner. But when our reason does not function according to the facts, in accord with reality, we are irrational (from the Latin root, *ratio* which means "reason").

I often hear the word "rationalize" used as meaning "to reason," (e.g., "I rationalized that it would be best to make my old car do for another year"). This is incorrect. To rationalize is to invent an acceptable reason for behavior that had its origin in subconscious motives considered unacceptable by a person. For instance, in the days when all women wore hats, a woman would buy a new hat and tell her husband, "I didn't have a decent hat to wear to my garden club." But actually she had been feeling very low and discouraged or perhaps resentful of what her husband had done, and had bought herself the new hat to get a "new lease on life."

Much less known is the fact that man possesses also a *receiving* source of knowledge which obtains its insights as free gifts, without the effort it takes for our reason to construct thoughts, judgments and solutions. Our intuitive mind (not instinctive mind) directly perceives truths independently of any reasoning process, but merely by, as the Latin root (*intueror*—to look, to view) indicates, by "looking," "considering," "contemplating." Our receiving, intuitive, or contemplative mind receives its knowledge from such sources as nature, the arts, faith and directly from God through the Spirit. If man can be said to possess a spiritual faculty, it is his intuitive mind that is at the basis of his spiritual life, and provides the link between the material and spiritual worlds.

While the Latin word for our discursive mind, for reason, is *ratio*, so the Latin word for our intuitive mind is *intellectus*. It is composed of *inter*–"between," and *lectus* from *legere*–"to read." We see the connection in the following example. You receive a letter from your friend after he has moved to another part of the country. The letter is full of information about his new life, his new house, his job, etc., which indicates he is doing very well. Yet you have read between the lines that he is not as happy as he wants you to believe. You know intuitively something that your logical, rational mind has not told you.

Q. I am familiar with the word "intuition," but that we have an intuitive mind is new to me. I took some psychology in college, but never heard about it. Everything you hear deals with our reason. I suppose that our reason or working mind is of far greater importance than our receiving mind. Am I correct?

A. In the final analysis the very opposite of your assumption is true. This may sound strange, if not unbelievable, because we are surrounded by evidence of what man's reason has been able to invent, build, compose, and provide for us in terms of material well-being. The numerous accomplishments of our technology and incomparable scientific endeavors seem to directly contradict my contention that our intuitive mind is primary and must be served by our rational mind, not vice versa.

In a sense this claim is confirmed by the fact that most, if not all, of our mathematical, philosophical and technological discoveries had their roots in a sudden gratuitous insight received in a moment of quiet, while napping, or during the time between waking and sleeping, yes, even in a dream. But always in times when our reason was least operative, so that in those times of rational inactivity it was possible for the receiving mind to be receptive to previously unknown ideas and concepts. For sure, these novel ideas have to be developed and tested by the working mind, but it was the intuitive mind that received in its openness the *gift* of the novel idea. It is somewhat like our inability to recall a certain known fact no matter how hard we try, until we decide to stop all these efforts of our reason, and the result is that the answer suddenly "pops" into our mind.

There are two more reasons for describing our intuitive or gifted mind as superior to our reasoning mind. If you agree that the possession of a Cadillac is of a higher order than the hopeful expectation that you will have one some time in the future, then you must conclude the same for knowledge already possessed by the intuitive mind as compared with the knowledge yet to be arrived at by the discursive mind. You may counter that quantitatively the fruits of man's reason seem to far outnumber those of his intuitive mind. But this is not proof that reason is superior and primary to intuition. In our busy society, in which every person outstrives the next in the pursuit of happiness, our intuitive mind is simply not given sufficient opportunity to operate as it should. In fact, it is rusty from chronic disuse and will need much oiling and lubrication and patient attention in restoring its various parts to function, if we are to attain greater "mental health" than we have now in our sole reliance on our rational mind.

I am afraid that our interest in meditation and contemplation of the past decade will prove little more than a fad. Not because an answer to our need for happiness cannot be found there, but because Western people are always too much in a hurry to give a good thing like contemplation a good try. Unlike cattle that can be force-fed with growth hormones to reach the market sooner, or trees that can be made to grow faster and get to the lumberyards earlier, the activity of our intuitive mind cannot be speeded up by gurus or drugs. But more about this under the topic of "affirming living."

The second reason for the relative superiority of the intuitive mind is found in the difference between the nature of the truths with which both minds are concerned. Scientific truths concern our reason. Their discoveries can bring much happiness through greater material well-being. But our intuitive mind is the receptacle of spiritual truths, of things that lie beyond our senses and rational observation. These truths give us happiness of a higher order because they deal with more important topics than worldly things, worthwhile as they are. They are of passing interest to us. Not so, however, with the things not of this world, the immaterial or spiritual things that never decay or cease to exist—God, the soul, life after death, eternity, and so on. These are of lasting interest to man.

A final remark on this topic, of interest for women especially. Over the ages men have usually considered women's ways of thinking as being inferior to their own. Paul even told them to keep quiet in church, and governments forbade them to vote. Their "emotionality" was considered to interfere with their reasoning capacity. However, women always have been known for possessing a more developed intuition than men. Therefore, women must be considered to have a superior source of knowledge than men.

I do not know whether this difference is peculiar to the difference between the natures of men and women. I am inclined to think so. But if it is not, it must have developed as the result of centuries of women being far less preoccupied with worldly and utilitarian things than men, of having far more quiet and peace at home and thus of living in an environment that promoted the sensitivity of their intuitive mind. This argument, of course, would also hold true even if woman's intuitive mind is by nature more developed. In either case, modern woman stands to lose her superior way of knowing when she succeeds in becoming as active and driven as a man in her striving for the right to think, live and work like men.

Q. Can you tell us more about the relationship between our emotions and our higher faculties? At least, between emotions and intellect, since you have talked already about emotions and will.

A. I trust you will excuse me for having expanded on the subject of reason and intuition. But it is a most important subject particularly because it is largely ignored, or omitted in the specialties of psychology and psychiatry. However, with these insights we now are in an excellent position to understand the proper and healthy relationship between the two groups of emotions and the two kinds of cognitive sources.

Our receiving or intuitive mind is more closely associated with our humane emotions, while our working mind or reason exerts a greater and more direct influence on our utilitarian emotions. Our intuitive mind, with its knowledge of things spiritual, authentic goodness, beauty and truth, ennobles the humane emotions, which in turn enhance the intuitive mind's sensitive grasp of the personal, of relationships and intimacy, of love and friendship, of faith and hope. In fact, it is this ennobling influence that makes the emotions of the pleasure appetite truly human; hence my term "humane emotions."

When we speak of "knowing with our hearts," "heart knowledge"—the heart being the symbol of our emotions—we refer to the knowledge resulting from the interplay between our humane emotions and our contemplative mind. We cannot possess the full truth of anything unless we know it on both the intellectual and emotional levels of our existence.

Our reason and utilitarian emotions concern themselves with more mundane things, with the things of this world, with knowing and doing practical things, with effectiveness. Reason uses the psychic motor of the utilitarian emotions to compose and construct things, to achieve in business and to manufacture.

One can say that man's "heart" is made up of his humane emotions, ennobled by his intuitive mind. And his "mind" is his reason, aided by his utilitarian emotions.

A proper balance between our state of "affectivity"—our capacity to be affected or moved by our humane emotions—and our state of "effectivity," our readiness to think and act effectively, determines to a large extent our psychic wholeness, our maturity, our freedom from incapacitating psychic disturbances.

I shall say more about the interaction between our emotions and our higher faculties in later chapters.

Q. Is it true that love, joy, compassion, tenderness, empathy, sympathy, caring, appreciation of the good, the beautiful and spiritual truths, and all other emotions ennobled by our "gifted" mind, are the ingredients of the authentic happiness found in our

relationship with God, others and ourselves? And that our discursive mind, together with courage, hope, fear and anger, is involved in problem solving, technological achievements, overcoming obstacles, keeping safe, providing comforts and whatever else contributes to our material well-being and happiness?

A. Yes. But never forget, it is not a matter of either/or with respect to the distinctions I have presented in our emotional and intellectual lives, but a matter of both, each contributing in proper measure to the fullness of living. In every one of us there is need for a correct and continuously maintained interchange between the contemplative life and the active life, between intuitive and discursive activity of the mind, between being and doing, between being moved and moving, between "heart" and "mind."

Q. Are emotions purely psychic events, or are other parts of our being involved also?

A. Although the primary response to what our external and internal senses tell us about the goodness, badness, usefulness, harmfulness of the world around us take place in our psyche, there are always simultaneous changes taking place in our bodies. These physical, bodily or physiological changes do not follow the psychic event, called emotion; they are part and parcel of the emotion, and occur *simultaneously*. Thus we see here again another demonstration of the indivisible wholeness of our human nature, of the fact that we are "in-dividuals" (i.e., "in-divisible" units of psyche and soma). "Upward," the humane emotions are intimately linked with our spirit, and the utilitarian emotions with our reason. "Downward," both groups are linked with the bodily processes. It is through our emotions that psyche and soma are one. We are psychosomatic units or somato-psychic units. A change in the psyche produces a change in the soma, and vice versa.

For example, you can hear in a person's voice that he is very happy and excited, or you can see in the way he walks and picks at his food that he is depressed. Conversely, when someone punches me in the nose my anger may show in the color of my face and the trembling of my voice, or when I am told I have cancer my fear may reveal itself by my pupils becoming larger and the palms of my hands beginning to sweat.

The most readily observable physiological changes occur when our emotions of fear and anger are aroused. All of us are familiar with these changes either because we have felt them ourselves, or observed them in others. A more rapid heartbeat, sometimes to the point of palpitations; a flushing or pallor of our face; sweating; trembling voice; shaking of the hands or the entire body; difficulty in breathing; widening of the pupils of our eyes. If our blood pressure is measured it is usually up. Laboratory studies will show higher blood sugar levels in the blood, secreted by the liver to provide us with greater instant energy.

These simultaneous psychic and physical changes serve the purpose of enabling us to react in an integrated manner. If the fear of an attacker moves us to run for our life, the physical changes make this possible through the increased supply of energy from blood sugar, the increased blood circulation, etc. If our anger moves us to fight for our lives we are able to do this through this instant readiness of our body.

What I have said here about the emotions of fear and

anger holds true for all other emotions, although in some these physiological changes are not as pronounced and immediately evident to everyone. Yet, everyone is familiar, whether he knows it or not, with the effect of authentic love on the person's tender voice, touch, gaze and physical presence to the beloved. Compare this with the manifestations of selfish, sexualized love—the possessive kiss and grasping, overpowering of the other—and we realize how the emotion of love affects the whole person as a psychosomatic unit.

Recognition of these factors will aid us later in understanding why some emotional malfunctions make themselves manifest in psychosomatic disorders.

Q. Is there anything else we should know about emotions and their functions?
A. I cannot emphasize enough how absolutely necessary it is to always distinguish clearly between the emotion itself—the psychic arousal together with the simultaneously occurring physiological changes—and what is done in response to the emotion. Unless we clearly differentiate between emotion and behavior we will never overcome the confusion, fear and suspicion surrounding the topic of man's emotional life.

What you *feel* is one thing. What you *do* when you experience that feeling is an entirely different matter. We should also try to make this clear in the choice of our words. For example, what is meant when we say, "I became so angry when he called me stupid"? Did I merely feel angry inside myself, or did I also express or "act out" my angry feeling by slamming the door, raising my voice, blowing my top, swearing and throwing things?

We might possibly improve our communications by

saying, "I *felt* so angry when he called me stupid; but I did not do or say anything." Or, "I did not get angry," or "I felt so angry that I told him off in no uncertain terms."

Remember that the physiological changes accompanying a given emotion are *not* part of the behavior, of what is commonly called the "expression of a feeling," or the "acting out" of that emotion. These "expressions" or "acting out" go beyond the physiological changes either as "willed" or "uncontrolled" behavior.

The foregoing is beautifully exemplified in Ephesians 4:26, "Be angry, and sin not" (Douay). This means, go ahead, feel your anger, that is the natural way to feel when someone offends you. Then use your reason and determine on the most effective way to deal with the situation and the person who offended you. By doing this, and by not acting on impulse, you are able to refrain from a sinful action.

I shall come back to this Bible passage, and others like it, to demonstrate how it contains advice of great psychological value, in addition to its moral instruction.

Chapter 3

Fables and Delusions about Emotions

A *fable* has been facetiously defined as a "falsehood formulated to fortify virtue."

A *delusion*, a psychiatric term, is a "fixed false belief."

It is not an exaggeration to state that man's emotional life has been the victim, perhaps since time immemorial, but certainly in the last several centuries, of prejudice, fear, ignorance and half-truths. Though I doubt that anyone ever deliberately tried to mislead other people for the purpose of making them more virtuous, it seems likely that the emergence and perpetuation of many fixed false beliefs concerning man's emotions had its origin in misinterpretations of certain Bible passages and religious teachings.

It seems plausible to assume that other factors, too, have contributed to our present confusion in matters emotional—folklore, ethnic cultures, pagan beliefs, non-Christian philosophies and religions, etc.—but I have little first-hand information of this. What I do know and have learned in several decades of clinical psychiatric practice with a predominantly Christian clientele is the particular role certain pejorative attitudes and beliefs concerning man's feelings and emotions have played in the development of emotional-spiritual afflictions.

We should not hesitate to take a close look at this role provided we do so without blaming any particular Christian denomination, church or church persons, and certainly not blaming matters of faith and dogma. We desire to learn *what* is wrong, not *who* was wrong and responsible, directly or indirectly, for sufferings traceable to those misconceptions regarding man's "lower nature," his feelings, emotions and senses.

Q. Are you suggesting that the teachings of Christ as contained in the New Testament, and the teachings of the Old Testament, have been the cause of emotional immaturity and emotional illness?

A. Not at all. Those teachings, because of their divine origin, are unsurpassed in showing us how to live a moral life and do the' will of God. However, as the Bible is not a textbook of psychology, it has been possible for many to draw conclusions concerning man's nature that are not warranted in the light of what we now know. I presume that God did not consider it necessary at every point to inspire the biblical authors to write down things man could discover for himself in time by virtue of his intellectual acumen. And that is precisely what has happened even though it took many centuries to construct an intellectually satisfactory (comparatively speaking) psychology of man as man.

It seems to me that we have entertained for many generations a variety of mistaken notions about our own nature that have been detrimental to large numbers of Christians and Jews. Unfortunately, all new and current ideas about man's psyche and emotional life are not necessarily more sound than past Jansenistic and Puritan notions. In fact, quite a few of them already can be said to have an effect on people that is more disastrous than any of the old ones. In this century psychology, the study of man, his nature, and its powers, habits, and acts, is a strictly secular, scientific one, which tries to reach its conclusions independent of older, more philosophical approaches. Many modern schools of psychology seem to be totally unfamiliar with the insights provided in ages past, and thus handicap themselves unnecessarily in trying to know man in his totality. If in the past the investigative spotlight was focused almost exclusively on man's reason, will and spirit, and his "lower nature" taken more or less for granted, if not actually downgraded, the reverse is true in modern times. It was only recently that I read an article by a young psychiatrist, entitled, *The Reality of the Human Will: a Concept Worth Reviving*.[5]

Q. Do you agree with this suggestion?
A. Yes, I most certainly do. American psychology is an empiric science that views human behavior as a complex integration of basic biological needs and essential cultural adaptations, and determined by unconscious motivation. In focusing on man's behavior rather than his faculties, American psychology has proven itself inadequate in understanding man as possessing a spiritual dimension.

What is needed is a rediscovery of the philosophic foundations and supernatural premises of European psychology and Christian truths, to deepen our understanding of the clinical discoveries of American psychology and psychiatry. Moreover, the unearthing of some anthropological insights which have lain buried for more than seven centuries cannot but enhance this process of integration.

Q. Will you give us some examples of the misconceptions about our emotions that have proven to be harmful for the patients you have seen in your many years of practice?
A. Let me start with some general observations and attitudes toward man's emotional life, and then mention some specific examples. By the way, since the number of priests, religious men and women, and Catholic lay people I have treated in my practice outweighs the number of Protestants, my remarks will be based mainly on what Catholics learned as children in the home, school and religion classes.

It has always been a common practice to distinguish between man's "lower" and "higher" natures. This implied, of course, if it was not stated explicitly, that there was something inferior about our body, senses and feelings, and that only our "higher" nature—reason, will and spirit—could be trusted. The words "sensual" and "sensuous" always implied something bad and dangerous, almost as much as "sexual." The feelings and emotions aroused by man's senses and sex organs were considered to threaten and diminish his freedom to act in a morally correct way. In other words, man's "lower" nature was thought to have fallen more than his "higher" nature, whereas, in fact, his nature as a whole had been weakened or wounded by original sin (which left him also despoiled of his supernatural gifts of sanctifying grace, immortality, and integrity).

A commonly used word for "emotion," at least in the textbooks used by the young men in the seminaries studying for the priesthood, was "passion." "Passions" suggested something very intense and violent in the areas of sexuality and anger. They were mentioned in the same breath as ignorance as being enemies of our free will.

Young women aspiring to become religious sisters were constantly admonished from their first day in the convent to "rise above their feelings," and to ignore their emotions, if not also bodily pains and aches. Sensuality and sexual feelings were to be fought or controlled by will power and grace, if the individuals were to have a chance to become truly spiritual and holy persons.

A large variety of exercises were prescribed to help young men and women subdue their lower natures during the long years of training preceding ordination and profession of final vows. In nineteenth-century France a certain religious order of teaching brothers required their young candidates to use *poudre du pudeur* "powder of shame" when taking a bath, lest they would be able to see the submerged lower part of their body. (This order, like many other French religious orders, emigrated to America during the grievous persecution of the Catholic Church by bourgeois liberalism.)

In another order the members wore a metal chain around the loins directly touching the skin, which could be tightened when troubled by "impure thoughts and passions." "The third kind of penance is to chastise the body, that is, to inflict sensible pain on it. This is done by wearing hairshirts, cords, or iron chains on the body, or by scourging or wounding oneself, and by other kinds of austerities."[6]

In other religious orders the subjects had to rise from their cots in their dark cubicles during the night and at a given signal hit their bare skin with a knotted rope until blood flowed. In at least one very strict order of monks the men were required to sleep with their hands tied to a ring fastened in the wall above their heads.

These admittedly extreme practices are not recounted here for the sake of ridicule or cheap sensationalism, but merely to illustrate the deep-seated fear of man's lower nature that prevailed among Christians until fairly recent times. This fear drove the best of men and women to leave no stone unturned in "mortifying" (i.e., "bringing to death") passions considered hostile to their vocations. As these highly intelligent, God-fearing and well-intentioned men and women became—as priests, sisters and brothers—the educators of children and adolescents in generation after generation, the impact of this fearful attitude toward the emotions on the secular society was enormous. Because of the Church's preeminent position in the world this impact involved both Christians and non-Christians, aided and abetted by the contagiousness of the virus of irrational fear.

Thus teachers in Catholic schools, both religious and lay, either perpetuated certain mistaken notions about the harmfulness of particular emotions and bodily feelings, or they presented essentially correct notions in an atmosphere of fear and doubt that some pupils were unable to remain insensitive to. What these educators presented on the intellectual level was thus contradicted on the emotional level.

Q. But do you not agree that a certain amount of

fear is necessary to get children to do what is right so they will not give in to every feeling or desire?

A. I do not agree if it means making the child fearful or causes him to feel guilty for having a desire to, let us say, steal an apple. For man to experience the emotion of fear is proper only when he is exposed to or threatened by something potentially harmful. Though it is wrong for a child to steal apples from his neighbor's yard, the desire for the apple is not a threat; it is a natural inclination. The possibility of a beating if he steals is a threat, and fear of the pain may keep him from stealing. But the use of this threat should leave room for his learning to refrain from stealing because it is, in the first instance, the correct and desirable thing to do. Surely, for this his will needs to become strengthened so it can guide his desire in the right way. But we do not strengthen it by making children fearful of their emotions and drives. In fact when we do this we are setting the stage for a whiplash effect that will make itself felt at a later age. In time the irrational fear becomes an obstacle to the proper functioning of the will. (More about this in chapter 6.)

Q. Then how do we train children to do good and avoid evil?

A. The answer to that is that children are not to be trained in matters of morality. On this point the commonly held idea that man is a rational animal did not help anyone. Training is aimed at the correct performance of actions which may or may not be accompanied by a desire for doing those things. One trains animals to perform regardless of whether it is natural to them, or whether they like it. So it is all right to train a child to get up when the alarm goes off, to clean his room, to fix a broken toy, etc.

But in the matter of morals the child needs to be *educated* as to what is moral and what is immoral, and why this is so. With proper education offered at the right time—and this always varies from child to child—the child's love and desire for the good have an opportunity to develop, and likewise a dislike and aversion for the evil. And it is this growing combination of emotional liking and desiring the good, together with the will to do the good, that leads to true will power, and also to experiencing true joy in doing what is good.

Of course, this educational process requires much more knowledge and effort on the part of parents and educators; it requires much more than giving the child a licking when he misbehaves and threatening him with more of the same if he does it again. Moreover, the child needs the daily, living example of parents who live a moral life. This means that the child cannot be so readily left to the care of others—baby-sitters, day-care centers, etc.—for it is an individualized process requiring intimate acquaintance with each child's stage of development. To use some modern jargon: We have to know "where each child is at and where he is coming from," if we are to lead him to greater maturity. (This process is known as education.)

In essence, therefore, *moral education* makes every effort to safeguard the emotions against repressive influences so the will can utilize them, so to speak, in doing good and avoiding evil. It cannot be stated categorically that this has been true for past *moral training* methods.

Q. Thank you for setting me straight on the

difference between training and education. But I am sorry we got off the topic of past faulty notions regarding our emotions.

A. Let me now give you some examples of how it was possible for certain Church teachings, though good and correct in themselves, to become an obstacle to emotional maturity.

The Church has always taught that anger, together with pride, lust, covetousness, envy, gluttony, and sloth, were the "seven capital sins." They were called capital sins (from the Latin *caput*—head) not because they, in themselves, were the greatest sins, but because they were considered the chief reasons why men commit sin. Properly speaking, they are tendencies of our will to go against God's will in different ways.

It is not difficult to see how a child exposed at a tender age to this teaching could easily interpret his own feelings of anger, pride and envy as being sinful. (The four other words usually were beyond his comprehension and would not start to worry him until a later age.) As he was frequently not advised of the need to distinguish between the feeling of anger and the act brought about by the angry feeling, he usually would confess the number of times he had felt angry. Each time the priest absolved him of his sins the notion that angry feelings were sinful would become more deeply ingrained in his conscience. To this day many persons continue to suffer from a variety of ill-effects of these childhood impressions concerning one of their God-given psychic motors.

An essentially similar fate befell the notion of love. Failure to make the necessary distinction between the feeling of love and the will to love—willing the good of another person—has caused many a person to become guilt-ridden about his failure to live up to God's commandments to love God, parents, neighbors and enemies. Many came to hate themselves for experiencing feelings of hate and resentment toward an abusive parent, or a God who allowed his closest friend to die prematurely or innocent children to die of starvation or warfare.

The saying, "You must love your neighbor, but you don't have to like him," was one of the few attempts to help people realize that God's commandments did not concern themselves explicitly with the emotion of love, but solely with the orientation of the will. Of course, it was an inadequate attempt in the absence of a comparable saying concerning hate.

Hate, too, has an emotional as well as a volitional component. To feel hate for someone who always tries to make life miserable for you is a natural emotional response. It has no moral connotation. However, it is a different matter if one proceeds to will evil toward that person, to will his death, to damn him to hell. These acts of the will have a moral character.

Of course, one often made the distinction, "You may hate the sin, but not the sinner," but this did even less to prevent unnecessary guilt feelings—or even scrupulosity in sensitive souls—than the distinction between "loving" and "liking." I say this because, first, it is most difficult to make this distinction between sin and sinner in actual practice (one tried to *feel* love for the person while hating the things he did!), and, second, because ignorance about emotional and volitional hate deprived him of having certainty. It would have been helpful if one had reserved the word "hate" for the emotion, and "hatred" for the will-act.

The same comments apply to the "sin of desire" and the "sin of despair." The emotion of desire is different from the act of willing. Despair can only constitute a sin if the will assents to the emotion of despair thereby refusing to have faith in God.

Of course, we are familiar with the effects on children in past generations of grownups' attitudes toward sex, the air of mystery or taboo that prevailed in many homes, and the *over*emphasis in religion classes on the two commandments dealing with this topic. All this made it hardly possible for young people to discover that they could learn to be chaste and develop the virtue of temperance by means other than fear or emotional striving for holiness.

Q. Dr. Baars, much of what you have discussed about certain psychologically inappropriate presentations of moral truths has not been foreign to those of various Protestant denominations. Is it possible that these fear-inspiring teachings had a common root somewhere?

A. From talking with both Catholics and Protestant patients and listening to the comments from pentecostals and fundamentalists at my conferences and lectures, I have become increasingly impressed by the possibility that our common suspicion of our lower nature dates back to a certain interpretation of the story of original sin in Genesis.

In that account we read about Adam and Eve being tempted by Satan, and about their eating of the food from a tree that was pleasing to the eyes and desirable for gaining wisdom, which then led to their realization of being naked and filled with shame, followed by their banishment from the Garden of Eden. Through the ages, theologians have speculated about the precise nature of this sin of our first parents, who possessed the supernatural gift of integrity, i.e., the perfect control of reason and will over the emotions.

In the absence of a truly satisfying answer we usually have worked with the concepts of temptation, pride, disobedience, desires, nakedness and shame. It seems not too far-fetched to me to assume that in the minds of ordinary people "bad" desires and feelings could be construed to have been responsible for the sin of Adam's disobedience. Still, how could this be possible if Adam and Eve, before their sin, lived in a state of perfection of their human nature?

Although the foregoing is a pure philosophical speculation on my part for the fact that many Christians have a pejorative attitude toward their emotions, if correct it could explain why there are so many efforts in our day to discredit this part of Genesis, as well as other related Bible passages, and to present in their place evolution as a fact rather than what it is, a mere theory. To persons glorifying in our time the importance of emotions and feelings beyond reason, the story of the Fall represents a hindrance to their philosophy that man's feeling of love determines the morality of his acts (e.g., Situation Ethics). They prefer to explain the origin of man through evolution because this eliminates the biblical revelation that man, not God, is responsible for the evil in the world.

Q. Are there also other religious teachings that have been interpreted in such a way that it contributed to our past repressive attitudes toward our feelings and

emotions?

A. I suppose one could consider here those Scripture passages which for many have served as confirmation that the only proper relationship between the spirit and the flesh, between man's higher and lower nature, is one only of struggle and combat, not of cooperation and enlightened guidance. It is most regrettable that certain texts in both the Old and New Testaments, often taken out of context or simply misinterpreted because of insufficient knowledge of the beautiful way God has created man, have exercised an unhealthy influence on countless generations of men and women.

I shall quote a few of them to clarify what I mean. However, I do not want to imply that these passages have always been misinterpreted by everyone at all times. But because of what I have heard from thousands of neurotic Christians in my practice, I am certain that in some way or other they have played their part in preventing the emotional life from developing and becoming integrated with the rest of the personality.

I shall use here an older version of Scriptures (Douay-Rheims translation from the Latin Vulgate) because newer, modern translations are taking into account, at least to some extent, more advanced psychological insights of man and his nature.

Explicit or implied warnings against human emotions and man's lower nature can be inferred from, "When concupiscence hath conceived, it brings forth sin" (James 1:15); "Whosoever hateth his brother is a murderer" (1 John 3:15); "For when we were in the flesh, the passions of sins, which were by the law, did work in our members, to bring forth fruit unto death" (Rom. 7:5); ". . . and you shall not fulfil the lusts

49

of the flesh. For the flesh lusteth against the spirit: and the spirit against the flesh" (Gal. 5:16-17); "Let all bitterness, and anger, . . . be put away from you" (Eph. 4:31); ". . . whosoever is angry with his brother, shall be in danger of the judgment" (Matt. 5:22); "Be not a friend to an angry man, and do not walk with a furious man: Lest perhaps thou learn his ways, and take scandal to thy soul" (Prov. 22:24-25).

"Let not the sun go down upon your anger" (Eph. 4:26), suggested to some that one would risk dying in a state of mortal sin, if one had not confessed one's anger before the day was over.

In my childhood and adolescent years I was always led to believe that the first part of that same passage in Ephesians, "Be angry, and sin not," conveyed a certain association between "anger" and "sin." Only much later in my life did I realize how beautifully it expresses the proper distinction between the emotion of anger which is good and the consequent act which may be sinful.

The same negative connotation concerning anger was always implied in Jesus' teaching: "When a person strikes you on the right cheek, turn and offer him the other" (Matt. 5:39). No one ever explained to me that Jesus did not turn His cheek until His mission on earth had been accomplished and He had been nailed to the cross by His persecutors.

Until that moment of meek surrender had arrived He had always employed all reasonable means, when aroused with anger, to respond to every anger-provoking situation. For example, he used a whip on the moneychangers in His Father's house, and when He heard that His disciples had been unable to cast out the spirit from a possessed boy, Jesus replied, undoubtedly

annoyed, "What an unbelieving and perverse lot you are!
. . . How long can I endure you?" (Luke 9:41).

**Q. Are you saying that the foregoing passages
should be ignored because in some people they have
contributed to the development of a neurosis or
psychosomatic disorder?**
A. Not at all. Nothing in the Scriptures should be
ignored. They contain the words of God without which we
can never share in His happiness. Therefore, it is fitting
that we do whatever is reasonable to harmonize them
with the greater knowledge we now possess about the
beautiful way our Creator fashioned man. Modern Bible
scholars are doing their share by giving us better
translations. Wherever indicated they should be aided
by experts in the human sciences who are convinced that
there cannot be any discrepancy between our
understanding of man and what is written in the
Scriptures, and taught by tradition and the
representatives of Christ on earth. And if such
discrepancy seems to exist then exegetes and experts in
the human sciences should be able to come to a mutual
understanding that does not do violence to faith and
dogma.

**Q. What is your opinion about such expressions,
still used and heard to this day in religion classes and
the liturgy, as "The fear of the Lord is the beginning of
wisdom," "He will bless those who fear the Lord," and
the many other references to fear of God and of the
Lord?**
A. I am puzzled by the persistent use of these terms. It
seems inconsistent with the efforts of the Magisterium

(teaching authority of the Catholic Church) and others to make us more fully aware of God's infinite love, kindness, mercy and desire for man's happiness. The old images of a *wrathful* God ready to *punish* us with sickness and suffering in this life, and with hell in the hereafter, are fortunately making room for more reasonable accounts of God and the realities of evil, suffering and hell. But the use of the word "fear" in reference to God is, particularly for children, a reason to doubt His love and thus to keep themselves at a distance from Him. It creates in many a feeling of fear of something that is actually good. This, of course, is not healthy and becomes a ready source of emotional problems later on, if not of actual rejection of God and everything religious.

Most adults know that "fear of the Lord" means "reverence," "awe" and the like. But even those who possess this intellectual knowledge often continue to feel fear of God, if they have been raised in homes and schools—and have worshiped in churches—where they constantly heard God referred to as someone to be feared. A child lives predominantly on the emotional level, and for that reason cannot help but react emotionally with a feeling of fear to anything he is told he should fear. We do not do him any service by waiting until later to inform him that, according to Aramaic scholars, "fear" means "reverence." By that time the psychological damage has been done and will continue to plague him in spite of his "knowing" better.

Could it be that we Christians still have a long way to go in loving the Lord our God with our *whole* hearts? If we *really* had learned to love and trust Him wholly, one hundred percent, there would be no more room to fear Him, for "Love has no room for fear; rather, perfect love casts out all fear" (1 John 4:18).

Q. Is it also possible to get unhealthy notions about one's emotions without exposure to actual distorted teachings from religious sources?

A. Yes, indeed. A child may become afraid of his angry feelings when a parent gives him a beating every time he shows his anger. And when the parent himself is often unreasonably angry and easily provoked and makes the atmosphere in the home unpleasant with his moodiness, children often tend to suppress their angry feelings.

When parents quarrel frequently between themselves and hurt each other with their angry remarks, if not physical abuse, many a child resolves that he will never be like them when he grows up. He never wants to hurt others as his parents hurt each other when they get angry. Such a child then uses his emotional energy to repress first the outward show of his anger, and then the feeling of anger itself. He will have to suffer much because of this later in life.

Parents, teachers and other adults can convey mistaken ideas about emotions which cause children to stifle those feelings. Some of those ideas may be that "big boys and girls do not cry," that it is "childish and immature to get mad," that you "don't show your emotions in company," and that "only girls and women get emotional." The British have always entertained the peculiar notion that real gentlemen and ladies must be unemotional and in absolute control of their feelings. Their "stiff upper lip" and rigid, stiff, and formal relating to one another was the mark of class and refinement. Boys in England learned early not to complain for fear of being considered "sissies." In battle their deeply ingrained emotional suppression predisposed them also to great bravery by blind obedience to their commanders and their readiness "not to reason why, but just to do and die."

Scolding children for asking questions about sexual matters often creates feelings of fear, shame and guilt that become obstacles to the growth and integration of their sexual feelings. The same is true when the subject of sex is taboo and a hush falls over the conversation when a child happens to say something related to this topic. Of course, the "sexual revolution" has put a stop to much of this.

It is also possible that in spite of a healthy emotional upbringing an adolescent or young adult may suddenly start to repress his angry feelings and later in life suffer the consequences. I have treated several men for symptoms of severe tension (e.g., suddenly shooting a mirror full of holes, or attacks of angina pectoris on the way home from a pleasant and good job to a nagging wife) related to the time they had almost killed a friend in a fist fight in their late teens. These incidents had made them so intensely concerned about what their physical strength and anger could lead to, that they had resolved never to get angry again in their lives. This had become the beginning of a repressive process and the building up of tension-producing anger and resentment on the subconscious level. None of these men had been consciously aware of what they had been doing with their angry feelings and why.

Telling children that they are spoiled and selfish for desiring a toy or a pet, if in fact they are not, will also have a detrimental effect on the development of their emotional life. Instead of making the child feel guilty and ashamed of himself, and forcing him to stifle his natural desires, he should be told the truth, e.g., that the parents do not have the money at the moment, but hope to have enough when Christmas time or the child's next birthday comes around. In this way the child is encouraged to continue to desire and hope and daydream, all of which contributes to the total growth of his emotional life and its integration with reason.

Finally, I should mention another, very important obstacle to a balanced development of the total person—with the human emotions as the chief victim—namely the Protestant ethic of "work for work's sake," and "one does not work to live; one lives to work." From the days of the Puritans and Benjamin Franklin, a growing utilitarianism has eroded man's capacity for spontaneous enjoyment of life. As idleness had to be avoided because it was considered the "devil's workshop," opportunities for play and leisure were too little, so that the humane emotions had little chance to build a firm basis for a healthy emotional life. The drive to earn more and more money in the pursuit of happiness overstimulated man's utilitarian emotions, which further interfered with the need of the humane emotions to be the soul and center of man's emotional life. Happiness is not to be pursued or earned—it is a gift.

But here we are back again to the adverse influence of certain religious views of human nature. "For it was Calvin who viewed all pure feelings and emotions, no matter how exalted they might seem to be, with suspicion. . . . Thus Protestant asceticism turned with all its force against one thing: the spontaneous enjoyment of life and all it had to offer."[7]

Chapter 4

How Our Psychic
Motors Run

So much has been said and written about feelings and emotions in recent years that it would seem impossible to say anything on this subject that is not already known. Nevertheless, it can be done, and a great deal at that, for the simple reason that quantity does not necessarily mean quality. By and large current popular opinions about our emotions are rather superficial, if not off the mark. They seem to boil down to the belief that our feelings are all good and should never be repressed. There is rarely a mention of the difference between emotions and feelings, between feeling and acting, or between repression and restraint.

However, much more needs to be known about the reasons for calling man's emotional life good. Confusion in this area was and remains considerable. I see evidence of this every day in my practice and on my lecture engagements. Not even highly educated and intelligent persons—in business, professions, religion, education, etc.—seem to know what their emotions are all about and what to do with them. Yet without knowing why, they agree with those who claim that emotions are just fine and must always be expressed. They have no idea what is wrong with this assertion, or that it represents an overreaction to past unhealthy beliefs and exposes the pseudoscientific minds of those who proclaim this, and other equally wrong and even harmful ideas concerning emotions.

When these half-truths are taught by professional persons the consequences can often be disastrous. Some new syndromes of emotional disorders are already appearing among the many who swallow these novel concepts without prior chewing. Therefore, it is important, as well as urgent, that we begin to understand the fundamental principles by which our emotional life operates.

Q. What are these fundamental principles of operation?

A. In examining the claim that our emotions are good, not bad or to be feared, it is well to recall what I have said earlier about the need to distinguish between the emotion itself—the psychic awareness of the feeling together with its accompanying physiological changes—and the act or actions set in motion by the emotion, with or without the consent of the will.

With this absolutely essential distinction it is correct to say that each and every human emotion in itself is good because it is part of our nature which is created by God. And everything that God created and continues to create is, of course, good. But this goodness is a *natural* goodness, something that is good for us because it is fitting to our nature as man. We cannot say that an emotion is a *moral* good, for the emotion itself is not an act, and only acts can be said to be morally good or evil. Of course, in the past, Jansenistic and some other schools of thought implied that man's emotions were morally bad, and therefore many now overreact in holding that emotions are morally good.

When an emotion leads us to do something, and, of course, all emotions by their very nature tend to move us toward some kind of action, even if it is the decision to abstain from any external action, then what we do is subject to moral judgment. But the emotion itself never is. It is for this reason that no one can validly claim that what he did is morally right because "his feelings moved him to do this." This claim is most frequently made nowadays regarding the feeling of love. "When you really love, everything you do is right!" But what is "really"? And who determines what other motives for the action played a role in addition to the "real" feeling of love?

In other words, our emotions are good just as our eyes, ears, fingers and legs are good. All of them—emotions, brain, bodily organs, senses, etc.—are necessary for healthy functioning. And just as every bodily organ has its own specific function, so has every emotion. That we are not too familiar with the specific function of our human emotions is no reason to look at them askance, or to try to do without them as much as possible. Nor does it make sense to hold emotions responsible for immoral or antisocial behavior. After all, nobody blames the hands that steal, or the mouth that speaks offensive words. If hate leads to violence then it is because the person willed it so, or he was handicapped in controlling his response to the feeling of hate. We should see this as readily as we understand that a car is not responsible for a fatal accident. The blame must go to the driver, either because he willed the accident, or he lost control over the car, because of irresponsible driving. Or the manufacturer is to blame because he delivered it with a structural defect. Or no one is to blame because a tire blew out or some such thing occurred beyond the control of the driver.

Q. From what you have said it would appear that it does not make sense to speak of "good" and "bad" emotions, or of "positive" and "negative" emotions. Am I right in concluding this?

A. You certainly are. Our emotions are tools or faculties of our human nature which, when properly respected and used, aid us in living a truly human life. They contribute in their own way to our capacity for experiencing the happiness for which we have been created by God. It does not make sense to distinguish between "good" and "bad" emotions, or "positive" and "negative" ones. They are all equally essential, though, as I have shown, one group of them is of a higher order than the other.

If we had been told as children that our legs were bad and negative as compared to our arms, and possible sources of sin, those of us who were intent on living a good life would have become physically crippled by letting our fear suppress and perhaps ultimately eliminate the natural function of our legs. Of course, this was never taught and so we were spared the fate of becoming crippled and paralyzed. Yet, a similar thing was done in regards to our emotions, however innocently and blamelessly, and some of us have consequently become emotionally crippled.

Q. In spite of your explanations, I still find it difficult to see anything good and positive in the emotions of hate and despair.

A. I have heard the same concern expressed by many people in various parts of the world. Frequently they remind me that it is a sin to hate your fellow-man, and that it is a terrible thing, if not sinful, to despair. The word "hate" seems to be inseparably associated with "person," and when I point out that it is the same word as used in the sentence, "I hate rotten food," they immediately reply with, "But that is not hate, that is dislike." Dislike is a milder word for hate.

To see hate for what it is, a good emotion, it is necessary to distinguish between the emotion of hate and the will to hate (i.e., not to will another's well-being). It helps to compare these emotions of hate and despair with the feeling of pain. Nobody likes to feel pain, or is inclined to see it as something good, until it is realized that pain alerts us to the fact that something is wrong in our body and we should do something to right it.

When we feel despair we feel what at first we only suspected or knew. It is then that we are absolutely certain that a given situation is desperate. With this certainty, born of knowing and feeling, we are moved to try another solution or a new approach, in the hope that we can extricate ourselves from that desperate situation.

Let me add a few sentences to clarify the natural goodness of all human emotions. This claim pertains to all "pure" emotions, the eleven basic emotions I have described earlier, and named as such (e.g., anger), or with words indicating differences of degree (e.g., annoyance, irritation, mad, upset). It also pertains to words indicating a combination of "pure" emotions, such as compassion (love mixed with sorrow).

However, there are a number of words that seem to describe certain feelings (e.g., envy) which are not "pure" emotions, and therefore cannot be said to be good. Those "partial-feeling" words contain an element of willing or intending a certain action to follow the feeling. For example, the envious person desires something belonging to another person, and wills to deprive him of it if he has a chance to do so. "Lust" is another good example. It indicates that on the higher level one wills to gratify the sexual desire (which in itself is a "good" emotion).

I would advise the reader to subject all feeling-words to a careful scrutiny in order to ascertain whether one deals with a pure emotion, or not. This exercise will deepen your grasp of the meaning and importance of the emotional life.

Finally, it is necessary to realize that the high intensity of an emotion does not make it "bad," even though its consequences may not be beneficial for that person or others around him. For instance, anger that is not resolved in a reasonable manner grows into resentment or bitterness which can lead to a psychosomatic disorder, such as migraine headaches, and may manifest itself in a most unpleasant way to the people who must live with this resentful and bitter person. But this does not justify calling anger a "bad" emotion. What is "bad" is the failure to do something about the situation which caused the anger, and thereby letting the anger grow into resentment and bitterness.

It is also incorrect to say that fear is an evil, as I've heard some fundamentalists claim it is, because "Jesus told the people repeatedly not to fear." Jesus wanted the people to put their trust in Him, and to rely on Him to help them in all difficult situations which they were helpless to change for the better by themselves. Knowing our limitations, Jesus tells us: "When you are afraid and anxious, don't succumb to your anxieties—trust me, and I'll help you. Stop looking at the waves—look at me!" And "Fear is useless, what is needed is trust" (Mark 5:36).

Q. You seem to say we should own our emotions and focus our concern on how to respond to them in ways which will make our lives and relationships both happy and moral. If so, who and what determines what action we should take when a certain emotion has been aroused? And what determines whether that action is moral or immoral?

A. The answer to both questions is our reason. The better our reason is informed about the suitability and morality of the various actions that are worth considering in a given situation, the easier it is for us to act spontaneously. The suitability or practicality is determined to a large extent by experiences in similar situations in the past. The morality is determined by objective moral standards which every person, if he wants to live in an intelligent and responsible manner, must acquire through study and education.

Or, to say it in other words, our emotions need to be guided by reason. Persons who live in constant fear and worry let their fear determine what to do when they are desperate or depressed. Yet, it is not the task of emotions to interfere with one another, nor to control each other. All emotions are to operate on the same level, and reason alone can determine what courses of action are proper under the circumstances.

The next step is up to the will. One's will either abides by the information provided by reason, or ignores it and goes against it. Depending on whether the will is free, one's action is either morally right or wrong.

Q. But is it not true that our emotions oppose guidance by reason and prefer to go their own way? In the old days one often heard about the struggle between the flesh and the spirit; or that that spirit was willing but the flesh was weak. I believe that this referred to the struggle between the emotions and the will informed by reason.

A. Yes, emotions have usually been viewed as opposed to reason and will, and therefore were feared or considered with great caution and suspicion. Consequently, the emotions had very little chance to grow and remained in an undeveloped or repressed state, so that there was little for reason to give guidance to. A tour guide cannot be very effective if the tourists, in spite of looking like adults, are actually little children and prefer to do as they please instead of allowing themselves to be guided.

But this view is incorrect. This is not surprising, for it stems from a mistaken philosophy of human nature and human existence. Fortunately, there exists a more sensible explanation for the relationship between flesh and spirit. I discovered this during my search for a more sensible psychology and psychiatry back in the fifties when I realized that very few, if any, of my obsessive-compulsive neurotic patients responded to psychoanalytically-oriented therapy. Because details of this search have been described elsewhere, I shall confine myself here to an outline of the fundamental principles of our psychic motors.

It is important, however, that I give credit where credit is due. My colleague, Dr. Anna Terruwe, and I would never have arrived at a more sensible psychology if it had not been for some of the teachings of a member of the very same Church that I have shown contributed—unwittingly for sure—to so much confusion and unnecessary man-made emotional suffering. I am referring here to the anthropology (i.e., the study of man) of Thomas Aquinas, a thirteenth-century philosopher which enabled us to make certain clinical discoveries, which in turn prompted some Dutch scholars to reexamine the writings of this genius and doctor of the Church.

Much to their surprise these scholars learned that these writings about man, used by the Church for centuries as her official teachings, differed in some points from the original manuscripts. These manuscripts contained certain observations on human nature which were identical to or confirmed what we observed seven centuries later. We do not know why those observations were omitted but one could speculate that his secretaries or translators considered them so radical, that they were fearful they might precipitate a social and moral revolution by changing people's attitudes toward their emotions and feelings.

Q. What were those radical observations concerning human nature?

A. First of all, that man's emotions have an innate need to be guided and directed by reason.[8] That is to say that they need and desire to be guided by their very nature. Of course, this implies that this guidance could not be given properly unless reason first of all respects the emotions, listens to them, and accepts them for what they are—psychic motors that will provide the energy necessary for the many varied situations in which man finds himself.

The significance of this principle of the natural relationship between emotions and reason is that when an emotion receives its proper guidance, it is satisfied and is now disposed to submit to the decision of the will as to what course of action shall be taken. Regardless of what the will decides, the emotion will subside and lose its intensity until the normal equilibrium of calm that prevailed before the emotion was aroused has been restored. Let me illustrate this with a simple example.

I am strongly attracted by a member of the opposite sex—let us say a beautiful brunette—and desire to know her intimately. My reason tells me that this feeling of attraction or love, as well as my desire, are natural, because their object—the brunette—is a good created by God. Next, my reason—and faith—inform me, or remind me, that the gratification of my desire would be in direct conflict with my vowed commitment to my wife, and therefore a sin.

There are now two options for my will. I can choose to ignore what my reason—and faith—tell me, and will to gratify my desire. Once I do so my desire will subside, but I have committed an immoral act. More likely than not I will suffer feelings of guilt. On the other hand, I can choose to abide by what reason—and faith—tell me is my greater good, and renounce the gratification of my desire. In this case I act morally right, but more than that my desire will lose its intensity and subside. This it does because I have acted also psychologically right: my desire has been gratified, not as such, but insofar as it is desirous, in need of, rational guidance.

In our day people are so fearful of repressing their emotions and becoming emotionally ill, that this latter course of action is seen as a repressive act. That it is not, will become evident later when one understands the nature of the repressive process. In fact, in chapter 6, I shall describe how an obsessive-compulsive neurotic acts in the same situation mentioned above, and how his way makes it increasingly difficult for him to do the morally right thing.

As long as people do not know the difference between rational guidance and neurotic repression of their emotions, and do not want to become or remain neurotic, they are left with no other alternative than to express and gratify all their emotions. Unfortunately, however, the concept of rational restraint, i.e., not of the emotion itself, but of its possible consequent actions, is unknown to a large extent.

Q. You said this discovery was a radical one. To me it sounds very much like what we were told all along, namely, that our emotions must be controlled by reason. Are you not making much ado about nothing?

A. Your point is well taken. There seems to be no difference. But actually there is a world of difference. In fact, I am certain that if this radical discovery had received proper attention and had been taught in a clear and concise manner, our world would now be a vastly different one, much healthier, much less neurotic, more peaceful, more contented and happier. If past generations had had any idea that man's emotions are his friends and want and need to be guided by his reason, they would not have directed all their efforts and training methods at suppressing, if not completely eliminating ("mortifying") them.

It is true that we were taught that we must control our emotions by reason and will. However, this teaching often conveyed, if it was not explicitly stated, that, "You *must* control them, for if you don't, they'll cause you to sin; you *must* suppress your feelings at all cost; you can't trust them; if you don't mortify them—kill them—they'll get the upper hand."

Telling a child over and over, "You *must* control your emotions"—especially in an atmosphere that suggests emotions do not want to be controlled and guided by reason and will—creates an emotional climate in which the emotions cannot develop toward maturity and integration with reason and will.

Telling a child, "Your emotions *need* and *want* to be guided and directed by reason, and we will help you to bring this about by our own example and sensible teachings," enhances the growth of the emotions and their ultimate integration with the higher faculties.

The omission of this fundamental observation—and several other ones I shall mention shortly—from the masterworks of this thirteenth-century philosopher have cost mankind dearly. For centuries we have been wasting precious energy in promoting and enforcing a continuous battle between emotions and the higher faculties, instead of using this energy judiciously for the purpose of establishing an ever greater and ready state of cooperation and mutual support.

For countless generations the candidates to the priesthood were taught the above views of man in a rather dry, theoretical, nonpractical, uninspired way, because the heart of Aquinas's anthropological philosophy had been left out by assumedly fearful, short-sighted secretaries or translators. It is not surprising then that in spite of the fact that Aquinas became the official teacher of the Catholic Church, a contrary philosophy prevailed and dominated the attitudes and pedagogy of leaders and educators in the Church. It is this philosophy that was at the root of most of the practices I referred to in an earlier chapter, practices, rules and customs that led to much needless emotional and spiritual suffering.

Q. What is this other philosophy that is responsible for so much needless suffering?

A. I was referring to the philosophy—based, of course, on the belief that our emotions are enemies of our higher faculties and the spirit—which holds that man's will must be trained to act against his emotions, if he is to succeed in leading a virtuous life. This voluntaristic (from the Latin *voluntas*—will) philosophy, which considers the will as supreme, has dominated centuries of churchmen's attitudes and religious training.[9] For the past two centuries it was further encouraged by the teachings of the German philosopher, Immanuel Kant, who considered all human feelings as pathological. His ideas were responsible for such widely held beliefs as, "If you do something good when you do not like it and you *will* it with great effort and intense self-control, then your act is truly moral," and "What counts is that you *will* the good and do it, no matter how you *feel*."

As I shall explain in a later chapter, there is a direct cause-and-effect relationship between this belief that the will is supreme and must be exercised no matter how one feels, and the emotional afflictions of the scrupulous person, the obsessive-compulsive neurotic and instances of spiritual aridity of truly spiritual persons.

Q. What did Aquinas have to say about this voluntaristic philosophy?

A. Thomas Aquinas had some outspoken and well-defined views of this "will-philosophy." He stated explicitly that man's will was not the absolute and supreme principle of human conduct as was generally believed. The will, he said, was not to be trained to overcome and master our suspect and "dangerous passions," but rather to rule them democratically, i.e., to listen to them respectfully and together with them strive for the good. He called the will a "moved mover," moved by reason which shows us what is truly good, and moved also by the emotion of desire for that good. Aquinas evidently realized that all good, also and precisely the moral good, appeals not only to the will through reason, but also directly to the emotions of love and desire through the senses.

With this optimistic and positive outlook toward the value of a healthy emotional life, a person is able to strive for the good with two motors—those of desire and will. Such a person can be said to have real will power, because his will is supported by the desire for the good. This idea stands in stark contrast with the belief that evil has a much greater attraction for fallen man with his greatly weakened "lower nature"—or, according to some, with his corrupt nature—than his desire for the good could ever be. This attraction, therefore, had to be conquered or mastered by the will in its continuous battle between the flesh and the spirit.

The will had to be trained and steeled, for to "will"

meant to be in control no matter how one felt. It was believed that only in that way could one have will power. Actually, however, the will was trained and forced to do the moral good without the aid of the feeling of desire for that moral good. Clearly, such "forcing of the will" is inferior to the real will power that is derived from will and desire cooperating together.

Q. As Christians we are interested in leading a moral and virtuous life. How precisely do these truly new and radical notions of man's emotions help us to do this?

A. It has always been held that only the unrelenting training of the will could enable us to be virtuous. However, virtue consists of the habitual perfecting and ordering of the principles, the building blocks, of a human act. Since these principles are both will and emotions, and not the will alone, it follows that the cultivation of the emotions is as important as the thorough education of reason and the strengthening of the will in the development of the virtues.

And this is exactly what Aquinas explicitly said: "Virtue is not only in the will and reason, but also in the emotions." Cultivation of the emotional life in its entirety, not its extinction or repression, is a prerequisite for integration and cooperation between emotions, reason and will. The emotions together with their accompanying physiological changes exist in order to be ennobled and integrated harmoniously by reason, and thereby move us under its guidance toward the happiness for which we are created.

It hardly needs saying that this process of integration and cooperation is not an easy one and requires considerable time, at least the first eighteen years of life. Our fallen human nature with its imperfections needs all the help it can get from parents, teachers and spiritual directors. Jesus mercifully provided us with His Church and all her teachings, the Scriptures, the sacraments, and so on. Knowledge of the moral laws, philosophy, ascetical practices, etc., strengthens our mind and will. When we now learn to incorporate the whole of our emotional life according to the laws of our human nature, we will be in a much better position to live the Christian life. It is then that "the Christian ideal" can be really tried, something Chesterton said had "not been tried and found wanting; it has been found difficult and left untried."

What Aquinas said about virtue applies especially to the virtues of fortitude and temperance. Both require emotional involvement. In fortitude we are aided by the emotions of courage, anger and hate. A little reflection will make it clear that there is a big difference between the person who solely knows that something is evil and ought to be opposed, and the one who in addition also feels hate for that evil, is angry that it is corrupting or harming his fellow-men, and feels aroused to combat it courageously and vigorously.[10]

In temperance it is our desire for what attracts us which must be brought in ready alignment with our reason and will. This is beautifully demonstrated in differentiating between temperance and continence. Continence is the "minor virtue," for it consists of a violent and painful suppressing and holding back of the desire. It is a process that must be repeated over and over because the suppressed desire retains the same, if not steadily growing, intensity. This process of pseudo-control looks like the real thing because it is difficult, brave and energetic. It seems far superior to the ease with which the person, possessing the real or "major virtue" of temperance, directs his emotions.

Temperance, in contrast to continence, develops within the emotional life itself when the emotions are cultivated and given plenty of opportunity to run their natural course (i.e., to be accepted and respected and to be taken in hand and guided by reason). Because this is precisely what the emotions *want* to do, they become more and more responsive to and integrated with the higher faculties. In time there is an ever diminishing need for repeated interference by the will from without. In this way the emotions, and also such bodily feelings as desire for food, drinking, smoking, sex, etc., develop a habitual disposition to listen to their "master's voice," readily and effortlessly.

The temperate man, therefore, has true rational control over his emotions and bodily feelings, without stifling or repressing them. They contribute in no little way to his virtuous life. The continent man, on the other hand, has merely pseudo-control. His emotions have no part in his virtuous life. His moral life does not possess the joy and satisfaction the temperate man experiences.

Q. Aquinas must have been a real genius from what you have said so far. Did he also have insight into the nature of emotional illnesses, or did they not yet exist in his time?

A. There is no doubt about Aquinas being a genius. He received a superb education from his teacher, Albert the Great, a great scholar who did not confine himself solely to abstract knowledge, but used his journeys through the Western world to learn all he could about his environment through direct observation and experiment. He wrote two books, one on botany, and one on zoology. It was left to his star pupil, Thomas Aquinas, to establish order and integration in the tremendous abundance of Albert's knowledge together with that of Augustine, Aristotle and many others. Aquinas's greatest work, the *Summa Theologica*, was only an introduction to our understanding of God, man and all creation. To this day it serves as an unsurpassed basis of integration of man's new discoveries and insights by those who were so fortunate to be exposed to a true liberal arts education.[11]

Concerning your question about Aquinas's knowledge of emotional illnesses, I am pretty sure they existed in some form in his day. In fact, they must have occurred already in the time of Aristotle, the Greek philosopher who lived before Christ. After the new concept of neurotic repression on the basis of Aquinas's classification of the emotions had been formulated[12] some Dutch scholars researched anew the writings of Aristotle and Aquinas. It was then that they realized that Aristotle's terminology evidenced his knowledge of the repressive process as a battle between "overlying" and "underlying" emotions.[13]

Q. Can you give us a summary of the operating principles of our emotions?

A. Gladly. I will also add a brief outline of the two kinds of emotions and their functions. That way it becomes easier to see the whole picture.

1. Emotions are psychic motors producing motion and energy to make life easier for us.

2. The emotions of our "pleasure appetite," our "humane emotions," cause us to be moved. The emotions of our "utility appetite," our "utilitarian emotions," cause

us to move, to act, to do. Man's free will is the chief mover. Our emotions need to be subordinate to its direction.

3. Our humane emotions are intimately associated with our intuitive mind. Together they constitute the "heart." Our utilitarian emotions serve primarily our thinking mind. Together they constitute the "mind."

4. Our thinking mind together with our utilitarian emotions must operate in the service of our intuitive mind and humane emotions, not the other way around. Our "mind" must function in the service of our "heart."

5. All our emotions, in their "pure" state, are good and necessary for healthy living. There are no negative or bad emotions.

6. Emotions are natural tools with specific functions, precisely as our eyes, ears, hearts, lungs, hands, etc., are men's tools possessing specific functions.

7. All emotions have a need to be guided by reason and to be allowed to make their particular contribution to healthy living.

8. Any effort to interfere with the natural function of emotions will have adverse repercussions.

9. Every emotion is accompanied by certain physiological changes, which also must be recognized and allowed to be.

10. All emotions must be allowed to grow to full capacity and become integrated with and subordinate to reason and will.

11. Emotions must be cultured, educated and refined, so that they will respond readily to the will informed by reason.

12. It is not true that every emotion must be expressed or gratified (beyond the naturally occurring physical changes which are part of all emotions).

When the above principles are respected and adhered

to by parents and educators, the child's chances of becoming an integrated and mature moral person are much greater than they have been in the past. Nevertheless, because on this earth man will always live in the state of original sin (i.e., of imperfection) it will always be necessary to make many efforts to reach maturity. There will always be a need for ascetical practices, involving both pleasure and utility appetites, in order to attain self-control and unselfishness.

However, when the emotions are seen as integral parts of virtuous acts, instead of as enemies, the whole process of maturing will be much less painful and frustrating, and its successful end, other things being equal, will be virtually assured.

Q. You speak often of integration between our emotional life and that of reason and will. I find it difficult to form a mental picture of this process, both in its developmental and ultimate stages of completion. Can you help me understand this more clearly?

A. I think I can. Even if you have not grown up with a colt or filly, fed, washed and trained it, and have not become an expert equestrian, it would not be difficult to learn from the following analogy. Any person can develop a good image of the integrating process between emotions and reason and will, by drawing an analogy between the interaction of horse and rider, and that of emotions and the higher faculties. The horse represents the emotional life, the rider the life of reason and will.

The girl can hardly wait for the little colt to grow up so she can ride it. But she must wait for three years or so before the colt is strong enough. In the meantime she spends many hours with the horse, watching it play and run around, discovering itself and the world. She feeds it regularly, brushes its coat and patiently leads it by a rope around its neck. Thus they get to know each other, their likes and dislikes, temperaments, and other characteristics. They learn to respect and trust each other.

When at last the time comes to train the young horse the girl must learn this rather arduous and involved process from an experienced trainer. She is fortunate to find the best one in the business. She soon discovers it takes time and patience to teach the horse to go through its paces, to know what commands to give, how to bridle and saddle it, and many more things. The horse in the beginning tries to have its own way, refuses to obey, resists doing things that do not come naturally, yet responds little by little to the girl's gentle, yet firm insistence to make him do what she wants. Whenever the girl loses her temper and hits the horse, things get worse and the horse shows signs of obstinacy. The next day the girl finds it harder to catch the horse in the meadow. She has to be especially kind to regain the trust and cooperation of the horse. Both girl and horse, however, learn from their mistakes, and in time what was a struggle, and perhaps looked at times like a battle between girl and horse, becomes more and more a cooperative effort. After several years when the girl has grown into a young woman, and the colt has become fully grown and strong, everything goes smoothly because they respect and listen to each other. The young woman has learned to mount the horse as soon as she has fallen off. The horse no longer shies and rears as often as it did at first, while the young woman has learned to remain in the saddle when it does.

It has become a joy for the woman to go riding because the horse does all the heavy work, walking or galloping long distances, while she leads it where she wants to go with barely visible, but readily felt movements of her legs and hands. At last the woman and horse have become one, they understand and trust each other; together they do what neither could do alone. Through trial and error, learning from mistakes and successes, final integration has been achieved. With continued good care of the horse by the woman the daily ride is pure joy. She is free to let her thoughts and memories go out to whatever she wants. All her energies have become available for more important things in the deep satisfaction that she has become an expert horsewoman and free to go where she pleases because her horse serves her well.

Compare this picture of healthy growth and integration with that of a man who has always been afraid of horses, but who had to learn to ride one as his transportation depended on it. He had never fed the horse well in the belief that a weak horse would be easier to control. He had been most irregular in learning to ride it, for his fear of accidents had always been great. The more he pulled on the reins to keep the horse from going too fast, the harder it became to control it. Falls became more frequent as time went on. As the horse grew weaker and thinner from being underfed, the harder the man had to work to make it go where he wanted. He had to beat it with a whip to make it go faster, until at last the horse was no longer able to carry its rider. One day it lay down and died. The man had become exhausted from all his efforts to do things his way. He became seriously depressed with the realization that he had failed to train his horse in the way he had always thought was the best.

Chapter 5

Ecology of
Human Emotions

The word "ecology" has become a household word since so many people in our country have become concerned with the increasing pollution and spoiling of our environment. Ecology—from *oiko*, the Greek word for "house"—is the study of the relations between living organisms and their environment. Upon this knowledge are constructed the rules of proper management of the environment (economics), whether this be the home, a community, the state, the political body or nature. With proper management we avoid waste or extravagance, we save, we protect against spoiling, etc.

All this is applicable also to the emotions and the environment in which they develop. The immediate environment of a child's emotions is, of course, the parents and other adults. Their effect on the growth and integration of the child's emotional life is primary and far-reaching, for good, or for evil.

Q. I suppose parents, relatives and teachers should begin as early as possible in the life of the child to help him feel at ease and comfortable with all his emotions. Is that correct?

A. Absolutely. For parents and other adults who themselves feel comfortable with all their emotions and respond to them in mature and responsible ways, there is no special problem in this regard. They will automatically communicate to the child that his emotions and feelings are as much a part of him as his other faculties. Just as they do not tell a child that his arms are better than his legs, so do they not show preferences for certain emotions over others. Likewise, they will refrain from saying, "You must not feel sad, or angry, or hate," just as they do not tell him not to use a particular finger or leg. Yet, on the other hand, they will punish him for spitting on his little sister whom he says he hates, as much as for using his leg to kick a hole in a screen door. Just as they will help the child to strengthen his muscles through a variety of exercises and sports proper to his age, so they will help him to grow emotionally and to become increasingly sensitive and responsive to all that is good, beautiful and true, in ways that vary according to his age and unique personality characteristics.

They will be guided in this by the "laws of gradualness" and refrain from trying to accelerate the natural growing process of his emotions by giving him what is good too early and too abundantly. They will show him clearly and repeatedly why certain expressions of his emotions are harmful to himself and others, or self-defeating, inappropriate or immoral. The use of rational arguments, moral values, and their own consistently correct and moral way of living will be their main tools of educating the child's emotional life, reason and character. And finally, they will do their best to protect him from those outside influences that can damage the emotional development they have set in motion at home.

It is a different and much more difficult matter for parents and other adults who themselves have problems with their emotions. Their first task will be to try and correct in themselves whatever should and can be corrected. This book is intended to help them grow emotionally through new insights and to shield their children from the effects of what might be beyond healing in their own emotional lives. There is much they can do in this regard by simply refraining from actions, teachings, attitudes, etc., which are potentially detrimental to their children's growth toward emotional maturity. The parents' goodwill and efforts to learn what they can on this topic will pay off richly even when their own emotional health may not be as good as they would like it to be.

Q. Then the parents must begin to nourish and cultivate their child's emotional life from day one of its life outside its mother's womb?

A. Correct. However, it is even better if they start during the child's life inside the mother's womb from about the fourth month on.

Q. Are you putting me on? How can you influence the emotional life of a child five months before it is born? Or are you referring to its mother having regular prenatal checkups, refraining from smoking, drugs,

alcohol, and perhaps having a positive, happily expectant attitude toward her unborn child?

A. No, I am not putting you on. And I am not thinking of the prenatal practices you mention. They are all excellent and should be a part of her life from the time she knows she is pregnant. But there is a much more direct way of cultivating the unborn's emotional life, of making it really feel wanted and loved. When expectant parents follow my directions, their child will be emotionally much stronger and better equipped to deal with the tension and anxiety producing factors of our rather neurotic world. In other words, they can commence to promote their child's emotional health long before it first sees daylight.

Q. I can hardly wait to learn to do this. Is it very difficult?

A. It is a very simple way to communicate with your unborn child. Anyone can learn it easily and quickly. All that is required is that you are present to your child in a special way without doing anything. Just follow my directions.

A woman who is four-and-a-half or five months pregnant (or more) should gently put her hands on her abdomen, one on the right side of her womb, the other on the left. By leaving them there in the same position and without exerting pressure, she can cause the child in the womb to move from one side to the other. Thus she can gently "rock" the child from left to right and from right to left.

How does the woman do this? How does she communicate with her child? What kind of signals does she send out which can be perceived by the child?

What the mother actually does is nothing more than being present to the child in her womb with the full attention of her whole being. As she imagines it growing and living there in all its innocence and goodness, her feeling of tender love awakens and increases. If she wishes to touch and caress her child with her love, she can do so by letting her feeling of love flow into one of her hands, let us say the right one. In doing so she may or may not become more aware of the sensation of touch in her right hand as it gently rests on her abdomen.

Before long she will notice the child moving inside of her womb. It swims to that part of its temporary "home" where the right hand of its mother lies. The child nestles as it were with its back in the hollow of its mother's loving hand, somewhat like the little child does in the beautiful carving, illustrating the prophet's words, "See, upon the palms of my hands I have written your name" (Isa. 49:16).

When she now directs her feeling of love to her left hand, the child after a little while will sense this and swim to the other side of the uterus to nestle in the hollow of its mother's left hand. The mother "rocks" her child, swimming in the amniotic fluid, by a psychic process of extending her feelings of love now to one hand, then to the other.

How is this possible? In some mysterious way, but certainly not through pressure or change in temperature, the child senses this psychic force emanating from the mother, and responds by moving toward the spot where it enters its little fluid world. Mother and child give and receive in an interplay of love, a first for the child, months before it is ready to be born. The mother gives, and the child gives in return by actively receiving and responding to the mother's tender, but unspoken, sentiment: "It is good that you are here; I love to be with you; I love to play with you." And so the child "says" to the mother, "It is good to feel your loving presence; you make me feel wanted and worthwhile; it is good to be part of you."

That this exchange of love is most important to the unborn child becomes evident when the mother—and for that matter the father, too—has made it a practice to be present to their child in this affirming way every day at a certain time. If, for some reason, she skips one of these regular "visits," the child will react by kicking against the wall of its "home." It does not like to be ignored, and reminds its mother that it needs and wants to feel her love![14]

During the last weeks of her pregnancy the mother, in playing with her unborn child, can make it grow familiar with the birth canal, so that it will know which way it must leave the womb. During the process of labor and delivery mother and father should continue to be present to the child and guide it gently through the birth canal. Through this continued loving presence of the parents to the child the labor pains are considerably reduced and the delivery that much easier.

When the child is received on its entrance into the outside world with the same loving care and attention—in a quiet, semi-darkened, warm room, in gentle hands, without being slapped, but gently put on its mother's abdomen[15]—there is no interruption of the intimate bond of love between the child and its parents. It has a definite head start in emotional strength and bonding compared to the child who was never played with during the pregnancy and delivered in the more impersonal, routine way. With breast-feeding and continued good parenting, this child has an excellent chance of growing toward full emotional maturity.

Q. This is the best example of combined prenatal care and natural childbirth I have ever heard of. But now that the child is born, what is next on the program of training it in the best possible way to have strong and healthy emotions?

A. Just a moment. Remember what I said awhile ago about not using the word "training" in matters of morality? The same applies to emotional growth. I realize full well that almost everybody uses this word inappropriately, but unless we give up this habit, it will continue to interfere with our realizing our goal, namely, of helping people and ourselves to be healthier, more mature and integrated human beings.

In general one does not train human beings as far as their personal growth—intellectual, emotional, spiritual and moral—is concerned. Like animals, one only trains human beings to perform certain actions. One trains animals to be obedient, i.e., to behave in certain ways on command, regardless of how they feel at that particular time. This does not mean that one is insensitive to their feelings, or treats them cruelly. In fact the best training is done by means of rewards, rather than of punishment which makes animals obey out of fear. But even in reward-training one aims at the animal *doing* certain things even when it may not be inclined to do so *feeling*-wise at that moment. We train animals for our sake or convenience. We do not train them for their own betterment or "happiness."

It is possible to do the same with human beings. Superiors can train their subjects to be obedient for their own convenience. But this abuse of a superior position in which the subject is kept from maturing is a far cry from mature authority which demands obedience for the purpose of helping subjects to grow to ever greater emotional, intellectual and spiritual maturity. This, however, is an educational process conducted by already mature "authors" or "creators" of other human beings, not yet mature. It consists of leading or drawing out (from the Latin *educere*—to draw out) what is already present in an undeveloped state, with awe and respect and waiting upon, without forcing. It aims at an interior growth of emotions, thinking and willing that brings about the desired behavior.

There are exceptions to this basic rule. Military training aims at combat readiness to defend and attack under fire on command; the soldier's own life and that of his fellow soldiers depend on it. Persons who want to become pianists, surgeons, carpenters, astronauts, tennis players, etc., must be trained and train themselves by performing certain actions and bodily movements over and over again. The more and better they can perform these activities without thinking, the more effective and expert they will be in their occupation. Ideally this training process should complement, not be a substitute for, education.

Toilet training is an acceptable term as long as it is remembered that when the feelings of the child are taken into consideration the training process will have its desired effects quickly and without fuss. The time to begin toilet training is not the age stated in a handbook, or the age of the child next door when it was trained. The right time is when the child feels uncomfortable with his dirty diaper and wants to be relieved of it. This demonstrates the truth of all human activities, namely, that if at all possible, feelings should precede action. Only when this cannot be done safely and reasonably can training be instituted.

Q. O.K. I admit to using the word "training" in the wrong way. What is necessary to promote the full and healthy growth of a child's emotions?

A. I am glad you did not add "in the quickest possible way." Too many people are in a hurry for results in all their activities in life, even to the point that they try to accelerate natural growth processes. Everything in nature grows according to its own laws. This slow and gradual growth to a mature state must be respected at all times. It cannot be forced by man's hurried interference with the laws of nature. If, after a long, cold winter when one is eager to see the tulips bloom in all their beauty, one were to pull them up as they first break through the earth, they would be destroyed. When you force-feed trees the wood will be of inferior quality, less strong and too light. When you force a child to act as an adult before his age you prevent his emotions from maturing and enriching his life. I have treated many women for depression and being incapable of enjoying life, husband, children, and material blessings, because they always had to baby-sit with their younger brothers and sisters in their early years.

All one can and must do, whether one deals with plants, animals or human beings, is to provide the proper nourishment and protection from harmful, growth-stopping factors. In humans it is important to promote proper emotional nourishment. Nature will then do its part under the most ideal circumstances. And you can trust nature to do its work correctly! It may be too slow for you, but then you should ask yourself why you are in a hurry, and then take steps to live at a slower, more balanced pace.

Q. What do you mean by "emotional nourishment"? Is it all the stuff people are talking and writing about nowadays?

A. Not really. Though it is very important that we understand what emotions are all about, this knowledge is not the emotional food itself. Nor is it contained in the varied techniques and methods devised to counteract deficiencies in emotional development.

Emotional food for you or me is actually the emotions of other people. What other people *feel* and share in such a way that it can be *felt* (in the literal sense of the word) by a child, is the emotional food for his emotional life. The composition and richness of ingredients will determine whether or not child will ultimately become emotionally mature.

Everyone knows that in order to develop physically a child needs to be fed the right amounts and proportions of carbohydrates, proteins, fats, minerals, and vitamins. If his intellect is to develop to its full capacity he needs to be educated by his parents and receive adequate schooling from competent teachers. His spiritual life will unfold to the extent that he receives religious education and is exposed to persons whose faith and moral lives are a source of inspiration to him. But for a complete and total development of his personality the physical, intellectual and spiritual food must be complemented by emotional nourishment. Emotional health food consists of the right amounts and proportions of humane and utilitarian emotions on the part of the adults in his environment.

Unfortunately, in our society youngsters are given a lot of unhealthy emotional food, just as their bodies are fed a lot of junk food. This emotional junk food can do as much harm, if not more, as the junk food available in the grocery stores, cafeterias and vending machines.

Q. Can you give some examples of "emotional junk food"?
A. Smothering love; conditional love; spoiling love; self-seeking love; pseudo-affirmation; irrational fear; excessive emotional striving; incongruity between what is felt emotionally and its outward expression; inconsistent emotional reactions that confuse others; excessive rage reactions to minor irritations and frustrations. The chapter on emotional malfunctions contains many more examples.

Q. You mentioned the need for prevention of "growth-stopping" factors. Can you elaborate on this?
A. One of the first rules of healthy emotional growth in a child is that one allows nature to take its course by never telling a child not to feel this or that emotion, or to feel like others do. As long as the adults in the child's life accept and acknowledge his feelings—and for that matter also their own—the child will escape the fate of feeling guilty for experiencing certain emotions.

This may happen when a parent spanks a child for throwing a tantrum, i.e., for throwing himself on the floor, kicking it with his feet, and holding his breath. (This kind of tantrum represents the emotion of anger more than a willed behavioral response.) Surely, the parent may be extremely frightened when he sees the child get blue in the face and try to bring him to his senses by giving him a spanking. But is the child guilty of any deed that deserves punishment? He does not do any harm to the floor, nor to himself. Sooner or later he will have to catch his breath; if he wants to go on kicking, his muscles need oxygen for this. To feel angry when frustrated is a normal emotional reaction for which he should not be made to feel guilty. By leaving him alone the child learns it is acceptable to feel angry and frustrated, and that he does not get what he wants by scaring the adults with his temper tantrum. He then has no other alternative but to think of some other course of action to get the adults to give him what he wants, or to abide by what they decide is best for him under the circumstances.

As long as a child is never made to feel ashamed or guilty for his emotion of anger and the adults always treat him fairly and reasonably, he will over the years build an ever bigger storehouse of memories of "angry responses," some of which will prove to be socially acceptable and effective in getting him the desired results, while others will prove to be unrewarding and futile, if not counter-productive. An example of the latter would be a case of a child having to pay from his savings for the mirror he broke in a fit of anger. The larger the number of varied experiences a person has built up since childhood, the easier it will be for him, when adult, to decide quickly what action is most likely to be effective when he is irritated or angry in a given situation.

As such an experienced adult does not have to waste precious energy in suppressing or repressing his feeling of anger, he is free to quickly scan his storehouse of memories of similar situations in the past and weigh the pros and cons of possible responses to the anger-provoking situation. He may decide on a certain response because it is likely to move the other person who has offended him to apologize. Or he may prefer to say certain things which can be expected to make it clear to the other, who has taken him for granted, to treat him with more respect in the future. Or, he may use the occasion to clarify certain issues between them. Or he may decide to remain silent and do nothing, not because he is afraid to "hurt the other's feelings" or be disliked, but because in his opinion it is useless to try and make the other see it his way or offer an apology.

If a Christian, such an experienced adult will use every anger-provoking situation as an opportunity to help the other to be a better Christian (by making amends, apologizing, asking forgiveness, etc.), or to better himself.

Q. I am sure you have more to say on the subject of anger, but could you first discuss additional general rules that hold true for all our emotions, especially in the growing years?

A. The young child should be exposed to a full variety of stimuli of his external senses and his imagination, because these are the primary sources for emotional reactions. For example, a child should be given ample opportunity to discover his multifaceted environment through touch, taste, seeing and hearing. The toys in his cradle and later in the playpen; the dolls and stuffed animals and building blocks; the sandbox, pets, other children, water, grass, flowers, etc., provide multiple stimuli for emotional experiences of joy, sadness, likes and dislikes, desires and hopes, fears and courage and anger, and so on.

In Montessori schools children are exposed to an even greater variety of sense stimuli which further refine their senses and thus increase their sensitiveness. These excellent schools are sufficiently known that I do not need to describe here in detail how they contribute to the growth of a child's sense and emotional life.

Storytelling at bedtime, or other quiet moments during the day, is an excellent means of stimulating the development of a child's imagination. It is infinitely superior to hours of TV watching which actually deadens the imagination. Nature walks, playing with animals, discovering the many beautiful things made by God and man, all this stimulates the child's sense of wonder and awe and appreciation. Parents and other adults should be careful not to destroy this sense of wonder which lies at the root of his desire to learn, to respect and protect all that is, and to restrain himself from destroying or harming things and beings. His ability to control himself as an adult depends to a large extent on the early preservation of the child's sense of wonder.

Children should be given ample opportunity to play with other children. This teaches them to feel comfortable with the emotions of others and to share their own. It will develop their sensitivity to the feelings of others as well as their own. The oldest child in a family is often the victim of the mother's need to have someone baby-sit with the younger children. When the oldest one has to do this continuously, he or she is often deprived of needed time for play and recreation. Later in life this utilitarian blocking of the development of the adolescent's humane emotions will make itself manifest in a variety of neurotic symptoms.

Q. You mentioned the need for the child to become sensitive. Is there not a danger for him to become too sensitive? And if so, how do you prevent him from becoming hypersensitive?

A. The popular use of the word "sensitive" is often confusing. "You are so sensitive, you cry at the slightest provocation," or, "Doctor, I take offense so easily—I wish I were not so sensitive!" are commonly heard statements. However, one rarely hears people say that they are glad to be sensitive, though they seem to recognize sensitiveness as a good quality when contrasted with insensitiveness. It is good to be sensitive, and responsive, appreciative, to all that is good and beautiful.

It is another matter when "too sensitive" means being easily irritated, annoyed, hypercritical, bursting into tears of anger and frustration, and so on. This is usually the result of interference of the normal growth of the emotional life, especially through neurotic repression. I shall come back to this later. But timely exposure, in moderation, to all that is good, beautiful and true only makes for healthy sensitivity and appreciation and respect. It is one of the characteristics of true maturity in men as well as in women.

A few more suggestions: adults must set good examples for the child in "dealing" with their own emotions. For example, a father has been provoked by the destructive behavior of his child. The fact that he feels angry is conveyed in the tone of his voice as he takes the child aside, tells him what he has done wrong, and what his punishment will be. For example, he may say: "It is all right to feel angry, Billy, when your mother calls you in for dinner and you must interrupt your ball game; but it is not all right to throw the ball through the open window and break the mirror. You will have to pay for a new mirror from your savings." Telling the boy to drop his pants and hitting him with a strap, a barbaric punishment still used these days, is out. It leaves emotional scars and sometimes also sexual difficulties (masochism) which are difficult to treat successfully later on in life.

Parents should never shame their children for feeling certain emotions. Even if this shaming concerns only a single emotion, their entire emotional lives will suffer the consequences. It stifles their spontaneity and endangers their sensitiveness, a most important quality in interpersonal relationships. Our utilitarian, driven society is badly in need of greater numbers of women and men who are consistently sensitive, feel compassion for the poor and the sick, are gentle and tender with children, and have retained their sense of wonder, all without feeling embarrassed. In the present struggle for equality between the sexes this sensitiveness that underlies our mutual respect and consideration is in danger of being destroyed.

Q. A little while ago you spoke of the need to "cultivate our emotions." Do you mean we should stimulate our emotions and those of others in order to make them grow? I couldn't see anything good in doing that deliberately to our sexual feelings.

A. "To cultivate" means "to improve or promote growth; to develop by education; to refine." It is the opposite of "to neglect" and "ignore."

The cultivation of our emotions does not mean we must purposely stimulate them, and certainly not stimulate our sexual feelings. These make themselves felt spontaneously like our other bodily feelings.

When we cultivate our garden, we provide the proper amounts of fertilizer, water and air, while we remove the harmful elements, like weeds, that would impede or prevent healthy growth of plants. We then leave it up to the plants to grow naturally. The same applies to our emotions. We do everything reasonable to enable them to grow at their own speed and become refined, so they will serve us best in their fully developed, refined state.

Let me illustrate this process of cultivating in regards to the emotion of desire. Various misconceptions on this topic are detrimental to mature development. The core of man's emotional life consists of the emotions of love, desire and joy. If this core remains undeveloped it is impossible to attain the happiness for which we are created by God. The reader who has difficulty with this statement is advised to ponder Aquinas's formulations on this topic:

"To desire to be happy is not a matter of free choice."

"Man craves by nature happiness."

"The will strives in freedom for happiness, although it strives for it by necessity."

"Happiness is that which the will is incapable of not willing."

At the same time Aquinas takes it completely for granted that no full happiness can be conceived without pleasure and joy, without rapture on the part of the physical, spiritual-sensual being which is man.

One of the fundamental reasons why so many persons lack the capacity to fully enjoy the good which is theirs stems from the fact that the emotions of love and desire did not have the opportunity to grow and mature within them. In other words, to possess a good is no guarantee that it can be enjoyed and make a person happy. He must first have a desire for it, and what is more, that desire must have had the time first to grow to its fullest intensity.

It is, of course, only right to ask why this should be so.

The answer is that every human power or faculty, if it is to perform a perfect act, must be adapted to its object. All human faculties have a material substratum either by reason of their *nature* (e.g., our faculty for vision has its material substrate in the eye and the occipital cortex—a group of gray cells in the back part of the brain), or as a necessary prerequisite for their *action* (e.g., our reasoning power needs the gray cells of the brain even though it is not a function of those cells themselves). It is this material substratum that must be gradually disposed for optimum adaptation of its object.

A few examples will show that this is true for every sphere of human life, whether in the vegetative, sensory or intellectual order. Physiological observations, for instance, have shown us that the maximum utilization of food requires a preparation of the digestive tract through the secretion of enzymes and other substances which metabolize the ingested proteins, carbohydrates and fats into their corresponding human elements. This secretion can be enhanced through external sense stimulation, for instance, by smelling and seeing the food, by talking about it, or by such appetizers as bouillon or a small amount of alcohol.

The same is true for the sense organs which must be properly disposed for optimal perception of their object. This process of gradual adaptation, of course, takes place not only in the growing child, but also in the adult whose senses, developed as they are for the normal perception of their object, require further special adaptation for more critical perception. Medical students, for instance, gradually develop more critical tactile perception so that when they have become experienced physicians they can feel physical irregularities which are imperceptible to the layman. They also learn to develop their other senses, for example their power of vision, by which they get the capacity to discern even the slightest variations in the physical appearance of the patient.

That this applies also to the power of hearing is evident when we realize we have to learn to hear music, and that we understand and recognize the fine points of a symphony only after repeated critical auditions. Again the same is true for the sense of taste, for we all know that there are many foods which we appreciate fully only after we have become better acquainted with them—have developed a taste for them. The principle in all these examples is the same: each sense must be adapted fully to its object, if its owner is to be capable of maximal perception and thus greater enjoyment of this more perfectly perceived object.

Man's higher cognitive powers are equally subject to this principle. His mind must be opened, so to speak, in order to be able to grasp truths. Our higher education, especially through the masterworks of Greek and Latin literature, prepares man's mind to enjoy beauty, order and harmony, and elevates him to a higher cultural level than all factual knowledge ever could. The study of philosophy does this to an even greater and more spiritual extent. By philosophy here I do not mean the study of the various systems of philosophy, but the study of how to penetrate to the nature of things, of trying to understand the essence of things. It is this study of philosophy that forms our intellect and enables it to leave accidentals aside and to discover fundamentals and principles.

What we have shown to be true for man's biological functions, as well as for his sensory and intellectual cognitive powers, holds also true for appetites. When man desires something, he does so because he has recognized it as a good. This desire acquires its greatest fullness and depth when he knows the object in as perfect a manner as possible.

It is the emotional desire that must be adapted in regard to the desired object. This desire must develop, grow, unfold and mature if one is to enjoy fully the possession of the good. This, of course, happens only gradually, for it takes time to come to appreciate and desire the full meaning of an object. An object does not immediately appeal to man's emotions to its fullest extent; he sees something beautiful, he wants to possess it; he keeps on looking at it from different angles and discovers new qualities in it; the object becomes more and more attractive in his imagination and dreams, and his desire becomes stronger and stronger, with the result that when he finally possesses it the joy will be so much greater and more intense.

Once this desire has grown fully, and possession of the desired object has led to the fullest satisfaction obtainable, the emotional life is ready to enjoy another object, for its capacity has been enlarged, its owner has grown and developed more emotionally, and is therefore capable of greater enjoyment of the things that constitute a good for him.

This does not mean that every emotional desire must be gratified. Man always remains a rational being, and as such can never find adequate satisfaction from an object that is not at the same time a rational good. On the other hand, what I have explained so far *does* mean that the growth and development of a desire must not be obstructed in an irrational manner, and that one must foster its natural growth in order to learn to appreciate emotionally, with one's feelings, the countless goods God has made available to us. Only in this manner does one show a fully adequate gratefulness for and acceptance of God's gifts to us.

The necessary, natural growth of the emotion of desire is obstructed in the neuroses as the result of repression or deprivation (see next chapter). It also will be obstructed when the desire is gratified too soon. This happens in the well-known process of "spoiling." When parents give their children all the things they desire as soon as they desire them, or even before they had a chance to desire them, the children become spoiled. They lose, or do not develop, the capacity to enjoy enjoyable things because they did not have the time to discover and desire their full value as enjoyable objects. The natural harmony between head-knowledge and feeling-knowledge has become disordered, or spoiled.

When a spoiled child is given a toy that would give joy to other children for weeks and months, he will not give it a second look before long, because he did not have a chance to first develop a desire for that toy. When a child learns that he cannot have a thing as soon as he desires it, that it takes effort and money on the part of the giver, and that it is a special occasion when he finally receives it, he appreciates and enjoys it because it has gained special value for him. Because his capacity to enjoy that thing has grown, he is now disposed to enjoy things of somewhat greater value more fully and adequately. Under these favorable conditions the child's desires remain automatically directed at the goods that are proper to his age and nature. But the child who gets too many, too valuable toys, too soon is never satisfied with anything that is a source of joy and pleasure for other children of his age. He is spoiled for the rest of his life. His emotions have been *blunted* instead of *refined*.

This process of spoiling is not confined to material objects. A child can also become spoiled on the spiritual level. This used to be a common occurrence. Catholic children were expected to attend Mass on every school day throughout the elementary and high school grades. From the first day of school they were trained to sit still in church without talking, with hands folded, etc. Because of the praise—and often better grades also—they received from the sisters because of their good behavior in church, they were led to believe this was all there was to religion. They usually became bored early in life with religious things, and the expectation and desire for greater spiritual things never developed. By the time they went to college and were free to do as they pleased, many stopped going to Mass altogether.

In this connection it is good to realize we also give too soon, and therefore spoil a child's chance to grow to emotional and spiritual maturity, by our unbending, inflexible insistence on adherence to the letter of the moral laws. Telling a child that a *sin is always a sin*, and that he must do exactly what the Commandments tell him to do, is tantamount to expecting him to behave as an adult. This premature, rigid application of moral principles and the resulting feelings of guilt deprive him of growing up emotionally and spiritually, of learning from mistakes, and of discussing these matters with trusted adults.

On the other hand, one also gives too early by insisting that *sin is not a sin*. By telling a child or adolescent that masturbation is never sinful, but always normal—because everybody does it—one suggests that the sexual feeling must be gratified without delay, that having orgasm is all there is to sex. One thereby takes away all perspective, and deprives the young person of the expectation of a healthier, happier, shared sexuality in marriage. Matters are made worse, as is only too common nowadays, by advocating sexual intercourse at any age. This kills the expectation that sexual relations in an atmosphere of unselfish love could bring greater happiness. One becomes blasé in the mistaken opinion that there is nothing more to marriage and life than one's own intense sexual pleasures.

The proper attitude lies, of course, in between these two extremes. One maintains and respects the moral norm, but allows for growth. One assists the young when they make mistakes and do what is *objectively* sinful.[16] This is done because one knows that man sins only when he chooses evil freely, and that in the young the emotions which have not had the time to become integrated with reason and will, are not yet free. They are still blind, and need the guidance of the morally responsible adult.

Q. Is it correct to quote you as saying that you advocate that all emotions must be expressed for a normal growth of the emotional life?

A. No, I definitely do not advocate the necessity of the expression of all emotions at all times. The popular idea that all emotions must be expressed is incorrect. What I do stress is that all emotions must be *felt* when aroused. This is first of all an interior, psychic process. Part of this process takes place also in the body, where certain physical changes accompany what one experiences on the psychic level. As long as you do not make any effort to suppress these physical changes, some of which are noticeable by the outside world, the emotion will express itself naturally and spontaneously. This particular form of "expression" should never be suppressed.

It is possible, however, to go beyond this point of nature's "expression" of the emotion, and this is what is usually meant by "expressing one's emotions." One can shout and rage beyond nature's expression of a red face, a shaky voice, an angry look in the eyes. One can wail, cry, and tear out one's hair when in grief, but this behavior goes beyond nature's emotional reaction of tears welling up in the eyes, sad facial features, etc.

It is up to each person to decide if and when he will go beyond the "natural" expressions of his feelings. This decision must be made in each situation according to a variety of factors—who is involved, what is at stake, the source of the emotion, social and moral factors. If your reason decides, not your fear, that any expression of your anger might well cause you to lose your job, then you will decide not to do or show anything. But this is not repressing of anger by fear as the neurotic does. It is guiding your emotion and refraining from all external manifestations by means of your reason and will. As long as you act this way, you will never suffer any psychological difficulties, for you provide your emotions with what they need and want, namely, guidance by reason. Thus there is a world of difference between *rational restraint* of the outward expressions of your emotion, and *neurotic repression* of the emotion itself. This is the difference between emotional health and emotional illness.

Chapter 6

Spotting Emotional Malfunctions

Now that we have a better understanding of what emotions are and what they are for, it is time to try to make some sense out of what must appear to many to be a bewildering array of neurotic symptoms and incomprehensible emotional disorders. Perhaps many professionals share this bewilderment, as there is now a movement underway to do away with the word "neurosis."

Yet, it is not too difficult to present a clear outline of those common emotional afflictions that concern all of us in some way. Whether we ourselves suffer from these afflictions or not, our entire society has an important stake in their successful treatment and their prevention in the future. In my opinion, the nonprofessional, the man in the street, will have to play an active part, whether as parent, teacher, educator, or in the increasingly popular area of "inner healing" by charismatics and pentecostals. Without the help of the nonprofessional, the psychiatrists and other mental health professionals can never hope to succeed in significantly reducing the incidence of emotional illness in present and future generations.

In order to gain a practical and adequate understanding of the most common, widespread emotional afflictions, it suffices to distinguish between the neuroses caused by repression, those caused by deprivation, and the nonneurotic conditions.

Q. Dr. Baars, before you start discussing the various types of emotional disorders, will you please explain the difference between such terms as mental and emotional illness or health, neurosis and psychosis, and other commonly used psychiatric terms that lay persons often find very confusing?

A. An excellent suggestion! Let me start with the terms "mental" and "emotional." "Mental," from the Latin word *mens*, means "pertaining to the mind, intellect, or reason." Strictly speaking therefore, mental illness is a disorder of the reasoning processes—thinking, judging, etc. This occurs typically in a psychosis or psychotic state (like schizophrenia, paranoia, etc., and those conditions in which brain cells have been destroyed). However, the word "mind" has come to describe virtually anything that pertains to the psyche, as opposed to the body, like thinking, feeling, willing, memory, temper, character, etc. Therefore, "mental health" means "soundness of all psychological functions." However, because nobody has ever clearly defined the concept of "mental health," I personally prefer the term "psychic wholeness," which allows for the inclusion of the spiritual element of man.

"Emotional" means "pertaining to the emotions or feelings, as distinguished from the thinking processes of the mind." I think this is an excellent distinction that helps clarify psychological functions and issues. As there is already too much fuzzy thinking and talking in the fields of psychology and psychiatry, I shall make consistent use of this distinction between "mental" and "emotional," between "thinking" and "feeling."

Thus a psychosis is an illness that affects primarily the person's thinking processes (though it secondarily may affect also the emotions); it is a mental illness. ("Insanity" is a legal term.)

A neurosis is an illness that is primarily a disturbance of the emotions (though the thinking processes may also be affected secondarily); it is an emotional illness (disturbance, disorder, disease). The word "psychoneurosis" is an old term for neurosis; it is no longer in use.

The terms "psychiatrist" and "psychologist" continue to be a source of great confusion. According to a study by the American Psychiatric Association, "The public defines mental illness as crime, violence, alcoholism, depression and schizophrenia, and considers that the province of the psychiatrist."

This, of course, is a distorted view of what a psychiatrist concerns himself with. Moreover, it is misleading insofar as these areas mentioned represent different entities. Crime and violence are forms of behavior; alcoholism is an addictive disease; depression is a symptom; and schizophrenia a particular order of the mind. According to the above study the psychiatrist would not concern himself with neuroses.

Psychiatrists treat persons who suffer from different

types of illnesses, involving mind, emotions and body—which are characterized by a large variety of symptoms and forms of behavior. Many psychiatrists *specialize* in certain areas. I confine myself to the diagnosis and treatment of persons with neuroses (with or without associated spiritual afflictions). I do this because in this area I have something special to offer that I would like to make available to as large a number of people as possible.

A psychiatrist is a physician with at least four years of specialized education in understanding normal and abnormal psychological conditions. A psychologist is not a physician; he has also studied normal and abnormal psychology and is usually an expert in giving and interpreting psychological tests. He cannot prescribe medications to the persons he sees in psychotherapy, nor is he trained to do physical or neurological examinations.

"Psychopath" and "psychopathic personality" are also sources of confusion. Both are older terms, no longer in official use, to indicate a disorder that is neither psychotic, nor neurotic. The current official term for this condition, which often resembles a neurosis, is "personality disorder." This change may be an improvement to lessen confusion, but continued recognition and labeling of a variety of personality disorder subtypes perpetuates this confusion.

There are several examples of how confusing these subtypes can be. A "schizoid personality" indicates a person with a personality disorder with features resembling those of a schizophrenic; yet he is not psychotic. The "obsessive-compulsive personality" stands for a person with a personality disorder with features resembling those of an obsessive-compulsive neurosis, yet he is not neurotic. The same applies to other subtypes: paranoid personality, antisocial personality, hysterical personality, etc.

I will later discuss the fundamental characteristics of the person with a personality disorder, regardless of the subtype, since it is essential that one does not confuse this person with a neurotic.

Q. Is it possible for ordinary people to understand what neuroses are all about? Should you not have at least a college degree for that?

A. Not at all. Any one with a high school diploma can understand the different kind of emotional disorders, how they originate and what their symptoms are. Members of my profession, particularly the psychoanalysts, have made things unnecessarily complicated with the introduction of such words as "ego," "superego" and the "id." I have stopped using those and similar analytic terms long ago and substituted common sense terms from the field of rational psychology.

Q. On what school of psychology are psychoanalysis and modern clinical psychiatry based?

A. This is a somewhat embarrassing question, unless you are already familiar with the many diverse concepts and formulations in the field of mental health and illness. This is never clearer perhaps than in a court of law, where both the prosecution and the defense can retain psychiatrists to examine one and the same defendant, and have them end up with conflicting, even diametrically opposed, opinions concerning the nature and causes of the defendant's condition.

To answer your question, Freud, the father of modern psychiatry, did not start with a particular view of healthy or normal man. In other words, as a physician who had specialized in neurology (the study of the nervous system), he did not subscribe to any particular school of psychology. He started with emotionally and mentally ill people and interpreted their symptoms in his own, often most ingenious, ways. But they often had little or no bearing on the actual functions of the psyche of normal people as they were known in Europe in Freud's time. Since then, clinical psychiatry has been influenced increasingly by animal, experimental, social and behavior psychology—and more recently even by pop psychology—while the philosophic foundations of European faculty psychology have been absent from the American scene for the past half-century.

Without ignoring—in fact, with positive incorporation of well-established clinical findings in modern psychiatry, this book is based largely on rational psychology and faculty psychology (i.e., the study of man as man, the study of man's psychic faculties in the light of what man has discovered over the ages about all of reality, including man's beginning, his Creator and his ultimate goal of existence). Of course, here I address myself mainly to one particular aspect of this study, namely, man's emotional life, for the simple reason that it has been and is the least known and most neglected part of man.

Q. Can you give us a simple outline of the various kinds of emotional afflictions that make people go to psychiatrists and psychologists for treatment?

A. People go to psychiatrists in the hope of finding relief from the symptoms of a repressive neurosis, or a deprivation neurosis, or a psychosomatic disorder, or a pseudo-neurotic reaction (also called situational neurosis). I intend to outline these symptoms shortly in such a way that almost anyone can recognize them and determine their cause.

People with personality disorders do not visit psychiatrists, at least not voluntarily. Only when they are in trouble with the law, and that happens quite often, are they seen by a psychiatrist at the request of the courts.

Self-affirming persons by and large do not feel the need to see a psychiatrist as long as they expect to be successful in their striving to prove their importance and self-worth. When they have climbed to the top of the ladder of success and realize that is not the answer to their real expectations, it is usually too late to seek professional help. Death by suicide often intervenes.

As it is important to recognize self-affirming persons and those with personality disorders, I shall include a brief description of both. But first, I shall describe the type of neurosis that may have its beginning on the very first day of the child's earthly existence, if not before. Following that I will explain the neurotic conditions that start around the beginning of elementary school and the neurotic-like conditions that originate later on in life.

When a child is deprived in infancy, childhood, or puberty of the most fundamental element of emotional nourishment, namely, the unselfish, mature love of an adult person, he remains incapable of experiencing joy and happiness. As long as this fundamental need for being loved for what he *is* (as distinguished from for what he *does* or *achieves*) is frustrated, he hungers for feeling loved and wanted, for having a sense of belonging, for being loveable, for feeling worthwhile and significant for being who he is, for being unique, yes, simply for existing.

The child's need for feeling loved is as fundamental as his need for food, air, and shelter. He cannot live if this need is not satisfied. Exist, yes, but not really live as a human being should live. Without this fundamental feeling of being loved by another being, he will continue to crave it. As long as this craving is frustrated, his emotional life cannot develop. By this I mean that he cannot develop that part of his emotional life that is primary—his humane emotions which, together with his intuitive mind, determine his happiness and his capacity of making other people truly happy. The other part, however, his utilitarian emotions, usually develop to excess—too much fear and despair in some, too much energetic striving in others.

His psychic birth, as distinct from his physical birth, cannot take place without the gratification of this fundamental need. Without this second birth he remains emotionally a child, even though his body, intellect and spiritual life grow, provided, of course, that these parts of his being are given the proper food. Usually his intellectual and spiritual lives will suffer, even though the damage may not become noticeable until much later, particularly in times of great crises. It is then that one realizes that such an emotionally deprived person is like a house built without a firm foundation. It collapses in a storm, and what looked like a beautiful and strong superstructure of academic degrees, great business acumen, political talent, or religious fervor proves to possess no real strength. Genuine strength is found in the "heart"—the humane emotions interacting with the intuitive mind—which cements the body to the structures of intellect and spirit.

Q. I am sorry for interrupting you, but you started out by calling this deprived condition a neurosis. Yet you have not talked at all of a repression of unacceptable emotions and feelings. I have always heard that all neuroses are caused by the repression of unacceptable feelings. Isn't that what Freud has always taught?

A. Yes, you are entirely correct in saying that Freud taught this. And what is more, the psychiatric profession as a whole still clings to this idea that all neuroses are repressive neuroses. Yet the damage to a person's emotional life which I just described is not at all due to repression. It is solely the result of adults withholding from him what is an essential building stone of his emotional life, of the infrastructure of the rest of his personality.

One of the reasons why this type of neurosis has been recognized so far by only a few psychiatrists is that some of its symptoms may also be seen in repressive neurosis, and even in people who seem to be "normal." However, when you see all or most of these symptoms in their "pure" state, especially when fully developed, as they are in what we have designated as deprivation neurosis, you will have no difficulty in recognizing it as a condition distinctly different from a repressive neurosis.

Q. Will every person who has been deprived of a parent's unconditional and unselfish love develop a deprivation neurosis?

A. Not necessarily. Every person who has been deprived of the gift of feeling his own unique goodness and loveableness is called an unaffirmed person. He has not been affirmed (i.e., strengthened by another human being). There are three possible developments.

First, if he was totally unaffirmed at a very early age of his life, the chances are that he will develop the symptoms of this condition to a pronounced degree. He develops a full-blown deprivation neurosis.

Second, if the lack of affirmation was not total, but only partial, and began somewhat later in life (or one parent made up to some extent what the other parent did not give at all), he is an unaffirmed person whose symptoms are milder and less pronounced. Many of these partially affirmed persons go through life as "normal" persons who are never really happy and content. Their symptoms are miniatures of the well-defined, easily recognized and disabling manifestations of the deprivation neurotic.

Third, if the partially affirmed person is by nature energetic, and has a lot of things going for him (e.g., a good or superior intelligence, the right connections, lucky breaks, a lot of money, a beautiful body in the case of women, and the like), he will often attempt to affirm himself. This means he will try to attain by his own efforts and means what he did not receive (or only partially received) as a gift from others. Clinically, the self-affirming person will appear and behave in a way that is totally different from the deprivation neurotic. Nevertheless, in close contact, a knowledgeable person will have no difficulty in detecting in him the same symptoms that, in more severe or milder degrees, are present in the other two types of unaffirmed persons, the deprivation neurotic and the "normal" appearing, unaffirmed person.

I shall outline the typical symptoms of the unaffirmed person, though only summarily, because they are dealt with extensively in my books, *Healing the Unaffirmed* and *Born Only Once*.

1. As the "heart" of the unaffirmed person does not develop, he grows to adulthood *feeling like a child*. He is fearful of the adult world, or the seemingly adult world, because many of his peers are also unaffirmed persons; he is lonely and afraid to disagree, to bother or displease others. As he bends over backward to be "nice," he ends up being just that, a "nice" guy, a "nobody" without personality or character, never standing up for anything he believes in, a person without enemies, but also without close friends.

When other persons lead their own lives and express their feelings without considering his, he feels excluded, left out, an outsider.

His only chance to establish rapport with others is to do it with his will. Superficial though it will be, it enables him to maintain his position in society. But as his willed rapport lacks feelings and spontaneity, it does not give him the joy of friendship and camaraderie.

2. As his childish way of feeling makes the unaffirmed person unsuited for the adult life he must lead, he experiences deep-seated *feelings of uncertainty* and *insecurity*. Even when reason tells him his willed actions and behavior in relation to others are correct, he lacks the corresponding feeling that this is so.

This explains why the unaffirmed person finds it most difficult to make decisions, hesitates to act and often changes his mind. This is true for interpersonal relationships, but much less in business or professional matters, which normally call for noninvolvement of emotional factors.

3. Because the unaffirmed person repeatedly fails in his

relationship with others, he develops strong feelings of *inferiority* and *inadequacy*. This may be manifested in the person feeling unloved, or ugly, or physically underdeveloped and weak, or even intellectually incompetent. These feelings are present in spite of the fact that the person *is* loved, beautiful, of superior physical strength and intellectual endowment.

In addition to these fundamental characteristics of every unaffirmed person, there are other symptoms that occur less consistently and universally. Their presence probably depends on a variety of factors: severity of the deprivation by the most significant persons in the life of the unaffirmed person, compensating factors in his environment, economic factors, relative intelligence, etc. To mention a few: feelings of depression; suicidal inclinations; feelings of guilt for being unable to love others and being self-centered;[17] impaired senses of touch, taste or smell; impaired power of observation; learning disabilities and impaired memory for concrete facts; lack of order and inability to discipline children or students, and physical and mental fatigue.

These and other symptoms are more fully discussed and illustrated in the books, *Healing the Unaffirmed* and *Born Only Once*.

Q. Dr. Baars, I cannot understand why the syndrome of lack of affirmation, or deprivation neurosis, is not yet generally recognized by your colleagues. It makes a lot of sense; there is nothing vague or mysterious about it. I do not think you have to be a psychiatrist or a psychologist to recognize a person with a deprivation neurosis. Are other psychiatrists and psychologists denying the existence of this diagnosis?

A. No, they are not denying it. They simply have not yet heard about it. They recognize, of course, its various symptoms, but not the sum total of symptoms as a well-defined type of emotional disorder with a precisely-defined cause and therapy. If they had, I am sure they would have taken some steps to list it in the official diagnostic manual.[18] This would be a boon for countless persons with emotional troubles, judging from the hundreds of letters I have received since we first published an extensive account of the deprivation neurosis in the English language.[19] Practically all write that they are amazed to read such an accurate account of themselves and their emotional afflictions. Many have added that they have been in psychiatric treatment for years and have never heard their doctors explain the nature of their illness in terms of deprivation. All ask for the name and address of a psychiatrist in their part of the country who understands their illness and can treat them accordingly. Having had to disappoint them in this request has been a source of much sorrow to me and them.

Q. Then why is it that your colleagues have not read your books? I read somewhere that *Born Only Once* is already in its sixth edition, and *Healing the Unaffirmed* is in its third. Surely the psychiatrists must have these books in their libraries.

A. Psychiatrists are bombarded daily with newly published books and articles. They have much to read and often insufficient time to keep up with their professional journals. Most stick to books by psychiatric publishers. When in the early seventies I submitted our 500-page manuscript for *Loving and Curing the Neurotic* to psychiatric publishing houses, I received nothing but friendly rejection slips and best wishes for publication elsewhere. I suspect that they did not feel comfortable with our occasional mentioning of God and the human soul, and topics like that. Speaking of such things is virtually taboo in my profession, even though psychiatrists claim to treat the whole man. But this whole man does not commonly include his spiritual life or his relationship to God, and life hereafter.

Therefore, when a nonpsychiatric publishing house happened to hear about the manuscript and offered to print it, we accepted that offer, even though we realized it would retard the acceptance of our ideas and discoveries in the psychiatric profession. In my opinion, it is only a matter of time before that happens. You cannot keep a good thing hidden forever.

Q. Are there many people suffering from deprivation neurosis?

A. Yes, there are. As far as I can determine, the number is steadily growing, perhaps even at an alarming rate. In our society the number of people able and willing to love their children and other persons in a truly unselfish and mature manner seems to be on the decline. This is not so strange when you realize that deprivation neurotics and unaffirmed parents raise unaffirmed children, who then deprive in turn their children in the next generation, and so on.

On the other hand, the number of repressive neurotics seems to be on the decline since people repress their emotions less and less. This is not as good a development as it sounds, as I shall explain in the eighth chapter of this book. Counting all unaffirmed persons—deprivation neurotics, unaffirmed "normal" persons, and self-affirmers—their number must be enormous. Have you ever noticed how many "normal" people are doing things because it is so "therapeutic"? They seem to sense that all is not well with them. "Mental health" in our society is at a premium; *psychic weakness* or *psychic debility* is all too common.

Q. Can you tell us more about self-affirmation? You make it sound like an abnormal and unhealthy process, yet I believe that some experts in your field speak about self-affirmation as a necessary step in one's psychic development.

A. It is true that some mental health experts, like Rollo May,[20] advocate self-affirmation. However, it is clear that they all do this without prior precise defining of "affirmation" in the specific psychological sense I have done. Therefore, their use of the term "self-affirmation" falls in the same category as "self-fulfillment," "self-realization," "self-assertion," "self-motivation" and similar not always precisely defined terms.

Self-affirmation, as distinguished from "other-affirmation," is indeed detrimental to a person's psychic health as well as to that of the people around him. Unfortunately, there are huge numbers of people in our society who attempt to affirm themselves, and have been doing so long before "mental health" experts began to promote this.

Self-affirming persons are unaffirmed persons who try to attain by their own efforts the feeling that they are good and loveable and significant, even though the important people in their early lives failed to give them that feeling. But the tragedy of it is that they never attain their goal. Even when they succeed in becoming very rich, or famous, or important in politics or business or the religious life, or whatever, and are envied or admired because of their power, and fame, they are doomed to discover sooner or later that they are still where they started from, namely, *feeling* unloved and worthless and insignificant. When people love and admire you because of what you have done or *do*, it does not mean that you will feel loved and worthwhile because of who you *are*.

Even though self-affirming persons present a totally different clinical picture than the deprivation neurotics, they are equally weak psychologically. They are both emotionally immature and weak as the result of not having been affirmed. The irony is that the self-affirming person in our society is even less recognized for what he is—sick—than the deprivation neurotic. He is usually thought of as mature, normal, yes, even above average. His effect on society is negative, if not destructive. He is incapable of affirming others, and frequently will not hesitate to use and manipulate for his own purposes the very persons who love him. But most of this is seen and interpreted as the "normal" behavior of the average American who is determined to get ahead in the world and give his children the material possessions he never received from his parents.

I am not saying that all men and women with their striving for achievement are necessarily self-affirming persons. As long as this striving remains reasonable and is not done at the expense of their children's emotional growth there is nothing to be concerned about. But the striving for power, success, fame, and the like, of self-affirming persons is not reasonable. Unless restrained by deep religious and moral convictions, as some are, they will not hesitate to work their way up at any price.

In my opinion, the growing number of reports of wrongdoing on the part of so many public figures in our society is a reliable indicator of the increase in the number of self-affirming persons. There is little doubt in my mind that there exists a cause-and-effect relationship between the growing incidence of self-affirmation and such new social phenomena and global problems as abortion on demand, the so-called sexual revolution, agitation for more equal rights and fewer obligations, pollution of the environment, monetary chaos and inflation, waste of food and energy, violence, and so on. I intend to write about this at another time.

Q. Is it true that if a child is brought into the world by truly affirming parents his emotional life is assured of developing to full maturity?

A. Unfortunately, this is not so. Even though that child has a definite advantage over those children who from day one are deprived totally or partially of authentic love, he can still be harmed emotionally.

Basically, this can happen in two ways. He can be made to repress certain emotions and thus begin to develop what later on in his life will be recognized as a repressive neurosis. Or he can be spoiled, as a result of which his humane emotions are blunted. Although this is not a neurosis, it will have harmful consequences for his happiness in later life. As I have discussed the topic already, I shall now explain what a repressive neurosis is and how it develops.

The deprivation neurosis, as we have seen, is the result of the child not receiving the proper emotional food of authentic love. A repressive neurosis, on the other hand, develops when adults give the child incorrect ideas concerning his emotions and bodily feelings which stimulate his utilitarian emotions of fear or/and energy. These emotions then begin to operate for the purpose of getting rid of those emotions and feelings which he thinks are bad, sinful, unacceptable to others, or cause hurt in himself or other people. The child may be informed correctly about everything else in the world, go to the best schools and so on, yet if he is given incorrect information, directly or indirectly, about the nature and function of his emotions, he has no choice but to react to this misinformation by repression, i.e., by pushing those emotions into his subconscious when he feels them. The same happens when he is given the right information, but prematurely, when he is too young to understand it.

How deeply and to what extent he will repress depends on several factors, both outside and within him. If the false information concerns the emotions which serve man's two innate drives (of self-realization and reproduction); if it is given earlier in life when the child's emotional life is not yet clearly differentiated; if the verbal misinformation is reinforced by nonverbal behavior, or if the correct verbal information is contradicted by the actual behavior and emotional reactions of the persons in authority (emotional junk food); then the repressive process will be stronger and its adverse effects more widespread.

If the child has an innate superior intelligence, if he is of a sensitive, serious and introspective nature, and sincerely motivated in willing to do what his parents and educators expect from him, his repression will be deep, consistent and, over the years, extend—by association or logic—to an ever greater number of sense objects and other parts of his emotional life. He develops what later will be diagnosed an obsessive-compulsive neurosis.

If the child, however, is of inferior, low, or borderline intelligence, not too sensitive or concerned about what he is taught, he will repress in a much more superficial way without growing involvement of other feelings and sense objects. He will develop in time a hysterical neurosis, with or without conversion symptoms.

Q. Are you saying then that in times like these, when every adult seems to be more or less misinformed about emotions and feelings, all children become neurotic, and develop either what sounds like a superior kind of neurosis, the obsessive-compulsive type, or the more inferior kind of hysterical neurosis?

A. It sounds indeed that there is no other alternative, and that one must expect all people who were born, let us say, in the past one hundred years or so, to be neurotic (even when not counting those who did not receive sufficient affirmation). However, even though I think that a large part of the Western world has been affected adversely by distorted beliefs about human emotions, I do not subscribe to the idea that everyone is neurotic or emotionally ill. There are always a certain number of children who let this misinformation go in one ear and out the other, if they heard it at all; or whose parents or educators for some reason just did not much bother talking about such things, and allowed their children to grow up pretty naturally and spontaneously—perhaps in rural, less sophisticated areas and times. The absence of emotional disorders in primitive societies suggests strongly that neuroses are the product of technologically

more advanced societies (though not necessarily
philosophically and spiritually more advanced).

Q. Can you tell us more about the manner in which
incorrect knowledge about the nature and goodness of
human emotions can cause a repressive neurosis? I find
that difficult to believe in view of the fact that Freud
has told us that it is the superego that causes a person
to repress. Your opinion seems to be quite different
from his and what the psychiatric profession in general
holds on this subject.

A. Yes, it is true that on this topic I am at odds with
Freud and those of my colleagues who still subscribe to
the idea that the superego is the culprit in the repressive
process. The chief reason for my disagreement was my
growing realization in clinical practice that if the therapist
was to correct, or change, or eliminate the patient's
superego which, the experts claimed, caused him to be
neurotic, he could run into problems of an ethical and
moral character (because the superego encompasses
conscience, moral standards and social mores). This made
me search for an intellectually more acceptable and
satisfying solution to the cause of these neuroses. I found
it back in the mid-fifties just as I was sufficiently
disenchanted to consider abandoning my profession. It
was a chance discovery during a visit to my native
country, but one which has brought me and untold
numbers of my patients much satisfaction and happiness.

Suffice it to say, in explanation of what I consider to be
the real cause of neurotic repression, that it is not what a
person *knows*, or *believes* to be true, about emotions,
human drives and human nature that leads him to
repress, but rather his emotional reaction to these beliefs.

His *fear* or *emotional energy* constitute the repressive force which moves him to try to get rid of feelings and ideas which he is led to believe are socially unacceptable, if not morally wrong. His emotional reaction does not depend so much on the actual teachings themselves, as on the emotional atmosphere in which they are presented.

For example, in the past, the sixth and ninth commandments often aroused fear of sex in children, not only because there were two commandments on this subject (while stealing, killing, and such had only one!), but also because many teachers couldn't help but communicate their own anxiety and discomfort with this subject. Other children, again, associated fear with the emotion of anger, and thus began to repress it, because they were hurt by their parents' angry punishments and beatings, or also because they saw their parents hurt each other in anger. These latter children commonly would decide never to let their own angry feelings be a source of hurt and distress to others, and thus began to repress their own angry feelings energetically, rather than by means of fear.

Q. Are you claiming then that a repressive neurosis develops because one emotion represses another emotion?

A. Precisely! It is not the superego—that strange concoction of conscience, moral standards and social mores—that forces unacceptable emotions into the unconscious, but another emotion that interferes with the natural course of an emotion deemed to be the potential cause of trouble. The child's neurosis has its origin in the intellect of the adults who must raise the child, and present it either with outright mistaken ideas about the child's own feelings, or with correct ideas before he is ready to understand them, or with correct teachings which are not further explained, or with concepts which are qualified in an atmosphere laden with fear, suspicions and doubt.

Actually these ideas presented by the adults have their greatest impact on what I have called earlier the child's "sophisticated instinct." Because this instinct functions in immediate, intimate connection with the utilitarian emotions, his response will be one of fear or energy (hope and courage). It is this emotional response which sets the repressive process in motion. Or, to say it differently, it is either the intellectual junk food fed to the children by the adults, or the proper intellectual food that is given prematurely and therefore cannot be digested properly by the child, that arouses his fear or energy, then and in the future, whenever these topics are brought up or personally experienced.

Q. Can all emotions function as repressive ones, or are there certain emotions that do this more than others?

A. Usually it is the emotion of fear that represses other emotions. Or, if it is not fear, it is the opposite emotion of courage (which for reasons of convenience we prefer to call "energy"). Both fear and energy are utilitarian emotions which in the normal person serve as motors that stimulate the person to protect himself from harm or to overcome obstacles. Like all other emotions they are good and necessary, but when they become engaged in interfering with other emotions they exert an unhealthy influence on man's psyche. This, of course, is because of the fact that no emotion should make it its business to prevent other emotions from running their natural course, which is to exercise their function in close cooperation with reason. All emotions should operate in equality, on the same level, and be open to the guiding or tempering action of will informed by reason.

In other words, the proper object of the emotion of fear is anything that is an actual threat to the well-being of a person, e.g., a rattlesnake ready to strike. And because no man has a single emotion that could be considered a threat to man, it is pathological to feel fear of another emotion. Conversely, the emotion of courage or "energy" serves the purpose of stimulating one to defend oneself against anything that threatens one's safety, health or life. Again, as no one emotion ever falls in that category, it is neurotic to use the emotion of energy for the purpose of battling other emotions. If one does so anyway, one will develop a repressive neurosis.

Q. Earlier you described how a healthy, mature person reacts to something desirable by giving the example of a man's response to seeing an attractive brunette. Would this be a good time to explain how an obsessive-compulsive person reacts?

A. When an obsessive-compulsive neurotic man—let us say, a scrupulous man—spots an attractive brunette, his immediate response will be one of fear. He is afraid she will arouse in him a desire that he considers sinful, potentially sinful, or an occasion for sin. He uses his fear to get rid of the desire immediately because he *wills* to lead a chaste life. He actually thinks what he is doing—letting his fear repress his desire—is the reasonable thing to do. He does not know any better, for he has grown up with this approach since an early age and his beliefs and actions are based on his *felt* interpretations of moral teachings.

But by repressing his natural responses to the sight of the pretty brunette—the emotions of love and desire—he makes these emotions inaccessible to guidance by reason. Because these repressed emotions are *buried alive*, and are not dead and forgotten even though it may seem so for the moment, they try to rise up in order to get what they need: guidance by reason. However, as soon as they get close to the conscious level, fear is aroused and pushes them back again into the unconscious. The *battle between fear and desire* is on, and goes on without pause, only to break down sooner or later in life.

Q. Is it as easy for a nonprofessional to spot a repressive neurotic as it is to recognize a deprivation neurotic? The fact that there are two different kinds of repressive neuroses, the hysterical and the obsessive-compulsive kinds, seem to make it more difficult.

A. Almost as easy, once he is familiar with the basic clinical symptoms that the obsessive-compulsive neurotic and the hysterical neurotic have in common. Then, when you see in addition to these common symptoms also the more specific symptoms of the two kinds of repressive neuroses—in the hysterical neurotic this could be a hysterical paralysis of an arm or leg; in the obsessive-compulsive neurotic this could be a hand-washing compulsion—then it is not difficult to make a diagnosis.

Q. What are the basic symptoms that all repressive neurotics, whether hysterical or obsessive-compulsive,

have in common?

A. The basic symptoms of all repressive neuroses are psychic and physical. The basic *psychic* symptom is that of tension. This is not surprising because in these persons two emotions are constantly engaged in a battle. Not just once in a while, but day and night. One does not repress one day, and deal normally with one's emotions the next day. The two opposing emotions are like the arms of two men engaged in arm-wrestling. The tension is as great as that of a rubber band being stretched between two hands pulling away from each other. Just as the band is under constant tension to the point of breaking, so the repressive neurotic suffers from a constant feeling of tension. He is constantly "nervous," tense, unable to relax.

As time goes on, this state of tension will proceed to restlessness, if not agitation, and an inability to sit still. Preoccupied with this tension and ways to find relief, it becomes increasingly difficult to concentrate on any particular thing. As the entire emotional life becomes affected in time by the repression of one single emotion, the person's reactions to stimuli from outside are increased and he becomes increasingly "oversensitive" and irritable. The smallest things bother him; he is touchy, jumpy, easily startled, and may at times "explode," just like the rubber band in time will snap. He is more and more "unreasonable" in his reactions to the world around him. All this, of course, is the result of the fact that the normal tempering and regulating function of his intellect on his emotions is being interfered with by the repressive process.

Because emotions have a psychic as well as a somatic component, *bodily* complaints also will make themselves felt sooner or later in the repressive neurotic. Most common complaints are fatigue, headache, backache, insomnia and some other ones, depending on individual constitution. The whole body may show the pressure under which the emotional life operates. The person's facial expression is often tense, while his posture may become bent or stiff. Not infrequently one can make a diagnosis of repressive neurosis by the way a person shakes hands; it is stiff and unnatural. Interestingly, the handshake of the deprivation neurotic is often the very opposite. It is often warm and prolonged as if he cannot or does not want to let go of the other person's hand.

Q. What are some of the more specific symptoms of the obsessive-compulsive neurotic?

A. Because in these neurotics the emotion that causes all the trouble, the process of repression, determines the clinical picture, we must distinguish between the fear neurotic and the energy neurotic.

In the fear neurotic the fear is so prominent that it places its mark on the entire personality. The fear pervades the person so intensely that it is aroused not only in the presence of an actual danger, like an approaching tornado, but even at the slightest possibility of danger, yes, even when no danger exists, but is only imagined. The fear neurotic lives in constant fear that danger may befall him. Because the true object of his fear—another emotion—is deeply repressed, or even better, *buried alive* in the subconscious, there is nothing the person can do to deal with it. Instead, his fear often becomes focused on all kinds of other things, which may or may not have a reasonable relationship to the fear. As the person is unable to do anything to get rid of his fears, his fear turns into anxiety. Every person who has suffered with anxiety knows what a dreadful feeling this is. It is especially terrible when there seems to be no way of getting rid of it. The anxiety is with you all the time and makes life a veritable hell. When this symptom is the patient's only, or most pronounced, complaint he is officially diagnosed as having an anxiety neurosis.

But usually, in time, other symptoms are going to develop too. Because it is most frustrating, if not maddening, not to know why one is so fearful and anxious, the mind will play a trick on the anxiety neurotic. This trick will give him the satisfaction of knowing, or rather of thinking that he knows the cause of his anxiety. Sooner or later the anxiety neurotic will find himself in an actually frightening situation, for instance, in an elevator stalled between floors. From that day on he will have a fear of being caught in an enclosed place—he has a phobia of being in an elevator, and of all situations in which he is not in control of the situation. At this point he receives the official label of suffering a phobic neurosis.

Typical examples of this kind of phobia is the fear of flying. I have treated several men who flew their own plane without trouble, yet were too fearful to fly in a commercial plane. Of course, the difference is that these men are in control of their own actions when flying their own planes, but not when a passenger in a commercial plane. These fear neurotics are afraid of the unexpected and are unable to trust other persons. The same holds true for people who are afraid to be a passenger in a car driven by somebody else. Others again have a barbershop phobia, and suffer unbearable anxiety when they finally must submit to the scissors.

It is evident to all that the life of a fear or anxiety

neurotic is far from pleasant. His life becomes more and more depressing. Whenever the symptom of depression becomes dominant he will be said to suffer of a depressive neurosis.

Because the repressive process is an unnatural one it cannot be expected to be forever as successful as it usually is during the adolescent and young adult years, when the fear is strong enough to keep the repressed emotion from surfacing. When the repressive process is finally beginning to show signs of wear and tear, the repressed emotion begins to sneak to the front of his awareness. The person then becomes obsessed with the very things he has repressed successfully for so long. If it was the sex urge that he repressed for so long, he now becomes obsessed with sexual thoughts, fantasies and so on.

From then it will not be long before he becomes compelled to do the very things he was always afraid of doing. For instance, he may now begin to masturbate or look at sexual objects. Though he experiences intense feelings of guilt and remorse when he does those things, after a while the compulsion to masturbate, or attend obscene movies, or purchase pornographic magazines will make itself felt again. If he is to resist this compulsion, he can do so only by virtue of a greater effort of the repressing emotion of fear, for his will was excluded long ago from dealing with the sexual feeling as it should. At this final stage the fear neurotic is labeled officially to have an obsessive-compulsive neurosis.

The difference between the official psychiatric diagnosis and mine is that the former is determined by the most pronounced clinical symptoms of the patient (anxiety, phobia, depression, obsession and compulsion, and some other ones I did not mention), while my diagnosis of obsessive-compulsive neurosis describes the nature of the illness and the kind of person who develops it (as distinguished from the hysterical neurosis). If it is fear that causes the person to repress I call this obsessive-compulsive neurotic a fear neurotic; if it is energy an energy neurotic.

From this brief presentation it is clear that the repressive process is always doomed to fail in the end in its purpose, namely, to do what one had been led to believe was right. This is a most tragic and frightening happening for the person who for many years had become convinced that he had it made as far as his control of his sexual urges was concerned. Having always conscientiously followed the admonishments, if not living examples of his educators who lived in chronic fear of everything sexual, he could not help but believe that his neurotic approach to his sexual urges was the only reasonable, correct and natural thing to do.

To experience this failure in one's forties or fifties after years of heroic practice of continence can cause many an obsessive-compulsive person to fear that he is losing his mind, or create an attitude of despair and self-reproach in the belief that he has lost his will power and succumbed to his "weak and evil nature." Of course, that person does not even know that his *will* had been inoperative in the repressive process, and that it is his *fear* that finally failed in its unnatural task of subduing other emotions and feelings.

Q. Is it correct to conclude from what you have said about anxiety neurosis that everyone who experiences anxiety is neurotic?

A. No, that would be a mistaken conclusion. Let me

explain what anxiety is all about. Many people are confused concerning this topic, which comes as no surprise when one learns that some psychiatric textbooks require three pages to define "anxiety"!

When our life, health, or whatever else we cherish is threatened by something evil, we experience the emotion of fear, which readies us, psychologically as well as physiologically, to defend ourselves or others. This we can do either by running away from the danger or, with the help of the emotion of courage, by opposing it in the hope of conquering it. In either case, provided we are successful, the fear abates. But what happens when we fail and thus remain exposed to the danger? It is then that our fear turns into anxiety, a most unpleasant feeling, but not necessarily a sign that we are neurotic.

Of course, the repressive neurotic is unable to deal effectively with the threatening evil, because he *does not know* what he is afraid of. He has repressed it deep into his subconscious, where it is beyond the reach of reason and will. Although in the beginning when he was young he knew what he feared, the ongoing repressive process buried it ever deeper as time went on, so that the whole process of repressing became automatic and virtually unconscious. Consequently, he became helpless in dealing effectively with what he had been told was a danger. His fear turned into anxiety along the way.

But it is also possible for a person to know exactly what he is afraid of, and yet not be able to eliminate it at will. This may happen, for instance, to a soldier in the jungle who is exposed to a deadly sniper he cannot see. If forced to remain in that jungle for a prolonged period, his fear may turn into anxiety—if not panic. This is one of the reasons why it is said that every person has his breaking point. The actor or after-dinner speaker may suffer enough anxiety to prevent him from eating. He knows what he is afraid of, but he can do nothing about it (except by being well prepared) as the time of acting or speaking is fixed.

Another possibility for a person, other than a repressive neurotic, to experience anxiety is when he *believes* himself too weak and inadequate to overcome what he considers a danger to him. A good example of this is the deprivation neurotic who lives in constant fear of the adult world around him. This unaffirmed person suffers from a fear that is not irrational, unlike that of the fear neurotic who, for example, fears invisible germs on doorknobs. Feeling like a child in the adult world around him is a *real* source of fear. His life is fearsome indeed. This *existential fear* disappears as soon as the adults become truly loving in their attitude toward him.

Once one is familiar with these two kinds of fear and anxiety it is easy to distinguish between them in meeting such persons.

Q. Awhile back you spoke of an energy neurosis. I have never heard that term used before. How can energy cause a person to be neurotic? I thought we were all supposed to be energetic and work hard.

A. Unless you had read some of our earlier writings you could not have known about energy neurosis. It is a new term introduced by my colleague in the Netherlands, when she discovered that a person could misuse his emotions of courage, hope, daring, or whatever you want to call them, just as much as the emotion of fear, and apply them for the purpose of getting rid of what are considered unacceptable or dangerous emotions, feelings and urges.

She decided to give all these emotions the collective name of "energy," as it is a fitting one in our energetic, driving and driven, aggressive and utilitarian world.

Of course, it is harder to spot an energy neurotic in this kind of world where the hard-driving, aggressive businessman is praised for his energetic pursuits even though it leads much too often to all kinds of physical and psychological troubles, if not to premature death from a heart attack. But this is all the more reason to recognize the energy neurotic early, because he himself is usually the last one to realize that he is sick and in need of help. Ordinarily, he does not come to the attention of a psychiatrist, except for such late complications as chronic alcoholism or depression.

Q. Are you saying that all people who are energetic are energy neurotics?

A. Not at all. Most of us need to be energetic in our work and lives. And even if one is too energetic and drives too hard part of the time or all the time, unhealthy as that may be, it is not sufficient to label that person an energy neurotic. The term "workaholic" would be more appropriate for him. It is only when a person uses emotional energy to interfere with and repress other emotions that he is neurotic. It is just like a person who is excessively fearful, scared of a little mouse or cockroach, afraid of a thunderstorm, etc. Unless his fear interferes with the natural course of his other emotions he cannot be called neurotic. Shy, timid, worrywart, etc., may be accurate names to describe that excessively fearful person, but not neurotic.

Q. How do you recognize the energy neurotic?

A. Characteristic for this illness is the all-pervading action of the energy that places its stamp on the whole personality. Although usually presenting an outward appearance of efficiency and self-control, the energy neurotic radiates an air of inflexible self-restraint that permits no natural spontaneity. He acts somewhat like a robot in the use of his will for the purpose of imitating the natural expressions of emotions: by smiling, laughing, looking sad, etc. He wills certain manifestations of emotions which he does not really feel.

He commonly displays an air of coolness and aloofness, even of hardness. The tension that is produced by the repressive process is revealed in his deportment and manner of speech, his tendency to overreact when irritated. In those moments his harsh, biting words, intolerance of opinion, and exaggerated outbursts are in marked contrast to his usual even, though always coldly polite, disposition.

Usually, energy neurotics are highly intelligent and gifted people who demand a repudiation of all feelings in everything they do, even in the spiritual life. Many even consider it their duty to rid themselves of feeling love of nature and art. Those feelings, they reason, might lead to the arousal of unacceptable emotions, and therefore should not be given an opportunity to grow.

Physical symptoms characteristic of energy neurotics are low or absent muscle-stretch reflexes, low systolic and diastolic blood pressure, and low or flat blood sugar curve. For these and other symptoms one should consult *Healing for Neurotics*.

Q. One often hears talk about hysteria and hysterical persons. Are those persons also neurotic, and

if so, what kind?

A. You are right in saying that the term "hysterical" is a common one. Unfortunately, though, it is not always used correctly. For example, people who wail at a wall, or tear their clothing at a funeral, are often labeled hysterical by people who grieve in more moderate, less emotional ways. As the word hysteria has no other meaning than "morbid, senseless emotionalism that is neurotic in nature," it is a most unfortunate choice of words, one that symbolizes the confusion in the minds of many about psychiatric topics. And this particular topic is doubly confusing, because there exists also the term "hysterical personality," to indicate a nonneurotic condition!

To bring some order to this topic that is confusing for most people, I shall explain these two conditions as follows. The hysterical neurosis is one type of repressive neurosis (the other being the already described obsessive-compulsive type). The hysterical personality, on the other hand, is one of many and varied types of personality disorders, conditions which have nothing in common with neuroses, other than their occasionally superficial resemblance. Since it is important not to confuse the hysterical neurosis, or for that matter any type of neurosis, with a personality disorder, I will describe the two conditions briefly.

Q. Why is it so important not to confuse these two kinds of conditions?

A. The main reason is that the hysterical neurotic can be helped psychiatrically, while the person with an hysterical personality cannot. I shall deal with this in the next chapter.

As I said earlier, the hysterical neurosis is caused by repression just like the obsessive-compulsive neurosis is. The difference is that *in the hysterical neurotic the repressed emotions are allowed to do as they please* and therefore will manifest themselves outwardly in the person's conduct. This differs radically from the obsessive-compulsive neurotic in whom the repressing emotions of fear or energy never permit this. In fact, the repressing emotions pursue the unacceptable emotions so relentlessly that they themselves, and not the repressed emotions, color the person's entire feeling life and conduct.

The reason for this difference is that the hysterical neurosis occurs almost solely in persons with a below-average intelligence, while the other type occurs in those with a superior intelligence. Consequently, when two persons with different levels of intelligence repress the same unacceptable emotions—usually sexual feelings or the emotion of anger or both—with the same repressing emotions—usually fear or energy—the less intelligent person no longer concerns himself with the repressed emotion once it has been made to disappear from consciousness by a single act of repression in childhood. The more intelligent person, on the other hand, continues to occupy himself with the repressed emotion in some way or other in order to be sure that it will never surface and lead to intolerable actions. The result of all this, of course, is that in the more intelligent person the *repressing* emotions of fear or energy dominate the clinical picture, while in the less intelligent one the *repressed* emotion will manifest itself without activating in any way the repressing emotion of fear or energy.

For example, if the sexual feeling has been repressed in a girl of below-average intelligence she will often act in a flirtatious way, while not having the slightest awareness of the fact that her behavior is "sexy" and suggestive of a desire for erotic affection or gratification. In fact, if a man were to take her up on what he perceives as an invitation for sexual intimacy the hysterical neurotic girl would turn him down because that is the very thing she fears.

Or a man may repress the emotions that serve his drive for self-realization, his assertive drive. In that case these emotions may make themselves manifest in a pathological need to be recognized, or a need to force himself into the forefront, perhaps in association with an over-sensitiveness to all kinds of real or imagined slights or irritations.

Q. What about persons with hysterical paralysis or blindness? Where do they fit in?

A. They fit right here. Although in general in the hysterical neurotic the repressing emotion (fear/energy) allows the repressed emotion (sex/anger) to do what it wants, it may at times become concerned enough not to permit its undisguised expression. When this happens the repressed emotion is forced to manifest itself via another route where the fear of energy of the person does not put any obstacle in its path. This gives rise to the so-called conversion reactions (the emotion is converted into a bodily reaction).

Such conversions may affect every area of the personality. When they affect the external senses, for example, blindness, deafness, tunnel vision (like looking through a tube), or insensitivity to pain may result. When the internal senses are involved the person may forget who he is (amnesia), or appear to be in a trance, or suffer fainting spells. Other hysterical neurotics may become partially or totally paralyzed in one or more limbs; or be unable to speak. Others again may vomit or have diarrhea without showing evidence of an organic cause.

But whatever organ system is involved in the conversion reaction, what gives away the nature of the condition is the fact that the person is not emotionally concerned about the particular somatic changes he developed. In other words, the hysterical paralysis or blindness, or whatever, is an emotionally isolated occurrence for the patient and lacks any identification with the repressing emotion. No wonder that the old psychiatric textbooks used to speak of *la belle indifference* (the "beautiful indifference" or "unconcern") of the hysterical neurotic person.

This must conclude my discussion of the emotional disorders called neurosis, whether caused by deprivation or repression. What is left is a discussion of a totally different kind of emotional disorder, because its cause is unrelated to repression or deprivation.

Q. I thought you were first going to talk about the hysterical personality and how he differs from the hysterical neurotic?

A. That is what I intend to do right now. But I want to make it clear that the only connection between hysterical neurosis and hysterical personality is the word "hysterical." They are *two entirely different disorders*. It is too bad that these terms continue to be used, because it causes only unnecessary confusion. As there is already so much confusion and disagreement in the field of psychiatry we should do everything possible to reduce it.

One way of doing this is by not concentrating on the word "hysterical," but on the question, "Does this person have a neurosis, a personality disorder, or is he basically 'normal' but temporarily acting in an overly emotional manner?" The question thus is, "How do we recognize a personality disorder, regardless of whether his subtype is hysterical, amoral, antisocial, hypomanic, paranoid, schizoid, passive-agressive, etc.?" These terms merely describe the main behavioral features of a person with a personality disorder. As these features may at times be seen also in psychotic or neurotic people, they could lead us astray if we focus on them, rather than on the underlying condition, called "psychopathic personality" or "personality disorder."

The three fundamental characteristics of a person with a personality disorder are as follows:

1. *Extreme selfishness.* Such a person relates everything to himself. His own self, and particularly his own physical and material well-being, is the only thing that matters. The good of others, if it means anything to him at all, always comes second. The psychopath does not know true love and friendship. If he loves it is only for his own sake, and the friendship lasts only so long as it is to his own advantage. In marriage the psychopath lives only for himself. The well partner is expected to adjust entirely to the psychopathic partner. There is not the least bit of devotion and concern for the other spouse.

2. In addition to this extreme selfishness, the emotional reactions of the psychopath are exaggerated, excessive, lacking in moderation (i.e., they are disproportionate to the stimulus). For instance, if he is slighted for some reason he may explode with anger, or show his displeasure for hours or days on end by a prolonged sullen silence. A

slight reproof at work may prompt him to resign on the spot. If in military service, a reprimand by a person of higher rank may lead to a refusal to obey orders or desertion. A scolding by a teacher may lead the psychopathic student to attack the teacher, and so on.

3. The immoderate emotional reactions and often impulsive behavior of the psychopath are accompanied by a marked lability of his emotions. Whenever his environment changes, or the sense object in his environment changes, his emotions change. A violent love may change to unreasonable hatred because of a trifle, and, conversely, a dislike may change into elation. His changes of mood occur not by the day, but by the hour. This is the reason why he is so unpredictable. One can never depend on him. His behavior is a constant surprise to others, and often beyond comprehension. As his emotional reactions and moods vary, so do his inclinations, interests and judgments, modified without any—at least for others—understandable motive. Often it is only a short step from excessive self-assurance and bravado to complete discouragement and indecision, just as inflexibility and stubbornness may suddenly turn into excessive pliability and dependence on others.[21]

Q. What are the reasons that psychopaths act in such a selfish and unpredictable manner? To me they seem like spoiled children who must have their own way at all times and don't want to share with other kids.

A. Unlike neurotics whose condition results from what their environment does to them, psychopaths are born that way. For some yet unknown reason there is a constitutionally determined lack of control of the emotional life by the intellect. It is as if there is a missing connection, or an unbridgeable chasm, between emotions and intellect. Both seem to operate on their own; each goes its own way. In that sense the psychopath resembles the animal who, because it lacks a higher life of intellect and will, reacts to what it feels impulsively, spontaneously, instinctively, or in a manner determined by its training by a human being. The animal reacts to the concrete sense object as such, while man, if he acts humanly, correctly reacts to the sense object only so far as it is reasonable to do so.

In the psychopath the normal subordination of the emotions to the intellect is not present, or only to a limited degree. For him the sense object has only sense value, and thus he lacks that which is precisely human in emotional activity. To give another illustration: a psychopath is discharged from prison after serving his second term for stealing cars. He knows that if he is caught stealing again he will get twenty years. Around the corner from the prison he sees a Cadillac with the key in the ignition. Seeing no one around he gets in and drives off, to be caught a few hours later. In contrast, the nonpsychopathic car thief gets out of prison under the same circumstances. He too sees a Cadillac with the key in the ignition. He does not drive it away, because he doesn't want to go back to jail. He may not have become an honest and law-abiding citizen but he is going to think twice before he steals another car.

Again, the exact cause of the psychopath's defective constitution remains unknown. It might be the result of heredity or of defective germ plasm caused by alcohol, drugs, etc. used by the mother during pregnancy.

Q. I have known some people who developed the

three fundamental characteristics of the psychopath only in later life. Doesn't that prove that this condition is not due to a defect of the constitution and present already at birth?

A. It is indeed true that healthy people can develop these symptoms later in life as the result of serious brain concussions, brain injuries by shrapnel, epidemic encephalitis (inflammation of the brain) or meningitis, (inflammation of the covering of the brain), and some infectious diseases of the brain. But this is not a reason to say that there is no such thing as a true or congenital psychopath. In fact, it makes it more likely that it does exist, for later in life acquired states of "pseudo-psychopathy" resemble the congenital ones so closely that they, too, could well be caused by somatic deficits in the brain, rather than by psychological causes. In my opinion, it will not be long before modern advanced research techniques will discover the exact cause of what some of us presume to be an organic deficit in the brain cells, or brain structures.

Q. Awhile ago you spoke of several subtypes of personality disorders, like the sexual psychopath and antisocial psychopath. Can you tell us more about these different types?

A. I can, but it is really not that important to know each and every possible subtype. It is just like cases of phobia. One can make a long, long list of phobias of this or that object of the fear, of closed spaces or open spaces, of heights or germs, and so on, *ad infinitum*. They may be interesting, but what is important is that one understands why a phobia develops, more so than what object is feared in such a morbid fashion.

The same is true for the person with a personality disorder. As long as we are able to recognize the three fundamental characteristics of this disorder, it is relatively unimportant how the individual psychopath's particular temperament, character and personality are affected by his constitutional organic defect. The danger of focusing too much on the subtypes is that one could easily come to assume that every person who manifests the symptoms of that one subtype is automatically a psychopath.

For example, a person may live in a world of imagined illness and believe himself to be suffering all kinds of ills, and, moved by a deep pity for himself, unconsciously exaggerates his complaints, thus trying to arouse pity in others. By focusing on this person's attention-getting behavior we may be ready to label him a hysterical psychopath, and thus untreatable, while actually he is neurotic, and thus amenable to psychiatric therapy. The same is true for the sexual psychopath whose sexual deviant behavior is one of homosexual activity. But this does not mean that all active homosexuals are psychopaths. Many homosexuals are neurotics.[22]

Q. Is this all we should know about emotional malfunctions?

A. There is one more item that may be of interest and practical help. It is the one exception to the rule that all neuroses have their beginning in childhood. Adults who have always been in good emotional health can, under certain circumstances, develop what is called a situational reaction, or pseudo-neurotic reaction. This will occur when a person deems it necessary, because of a new situation in his life, to repress an emotion, most commonly, I think, the emotion of anger. When he does so, he will begin to manifest the usual basic symptoms of repression, tension, restlessness, inability to relax and, in addition, often psychosomatic complaints, often followed by feelings of depression.

A typical example is that of the married woman who goes to the psychiatrist because of depression and/or considerable gain in weight. It is not hard to find out that these symptoms began to develop some time after her mother-in-law moved in with the family. When she began to make her presence felt with advice to her daughter-in-law on how she thought the meals should be prepared and the children reared, the patient decided to go along for the sake of "peace" in the family. This she got, but no inner peace. Her repressed feelings of irritation and anger gave her no peace. Her continued frustration drove her often to the refrigerator for some extra food, while her life became more and more tension filled. Depression followed.

Fortunately, therapy is usually successful in a short period of time, once the patient realizes what she has been doing and dares to break the vicious circle of repression, frustration and more repression. This is most easily done when she gets the cooperation of her husband whom she has been protecting from unpleasant relationships with his mother. A few talks by both with the house guest in which certain rules of conduct are laid down usually suffice to resolve the silent battle and its resulting repression. The depression clears up in a short time, and the extra weight is lost. Of course, the shorter the interval between the start of the repression and the time professional help is sought, the more rapidly the symptoms are relieved. It will take longer if many years have elapsed and the repression is chronic. Yet even here, because of the basic sound personality structure and preexisting emotional integration, the therapy takes effect much more rapidly than in persons who have repressed since early childhood.

Q. If I recall correctly, you mentioned earlier that psychosomatic disorders also fall under the heading of emotional afflictions. Can you address yourself to this kind of emotional disorder?

A. The connection between such psychosomatic disorders, as stomach ulcer, migraine, hypertension, dermatitis, and many, many others, is more readily understood when you recall that every emotion is accompanied by certain physiological changes. When a person represses a certain emotion, let us say anger, this emotion is prevented from being guided by reason. In other words, the anger is prevented from running its natural course so that it cannot quiet down and allow the peace and harmony of the emotional life to be restored. As I explained earlier, the emotion of anger is buried alive in this repressive process in the subconscious. Even though the person may no longer be consciously aware of his anger, it remains active, no matter how deeply it has been buried. But so do the various physiological changes that are part and parcel of the emotion of anger.

Some of these changes occur in the blood vessels of the heart and the body for the purpose of preparing the person to react efficiently to the cause of his anger. Once the healthy person has done so, his anger abates and the physiological changes in the blood vessels disappear. The anger has served its purpose under the guidance of the person's reason. All is well.

Not so, however, in the person who represses his angry feeling. The changes in the blood vessels continue as long as the anger remains repressed. In time they permanently affect the blood vessels and thus lead to such conditions as hypertension, heart attack or migraine. Bodily organs have become the victims of a psychic occurrence because of the physiological changes that accompany the emotions which constitute the link between psyche and body. A psychosomatic illness is usually a late development in a longstanding repressive way of dealing with a certain emotion. As any organ or organ-system can be involved, the literature on this topic is extensive. For the purposes of this book it suffices that the reader is familiar with the fundamental mechanism responsible for a psychosomatic disorder. This is particularly important for those engaged in the ministry of healing through prayer. In praying for healing of a physical illness they must not neglect to pray for the healing of the psychological afflictions underlying the physical illness.

Q. Dr. Baars, several times you have mentioned depression. You said it can be a symptom in the unaffirmed person, especially the deprivation neurotic, in a repressive neurosis, and just now again in the pseudo-neurotic reactions. But usually I hear or read that people suffer from a depression. This sounds to me that depression is an illness, not just a symptom.

A. It is true that both professionals and non-professionals usually speak of a depression, as if it were an illness in and by itself. Nevertheless, I believe there are good reasons to see depression most of the time primarily as a symptom that may be precipitated by different causes and in different situations. For instance, in a woman the change of life may cause "involutional melancholia," an illness in which a deep feeling of depression is the main symptom; a person who has repressed his feelings of anger from early childhood often develops a "depressive neurosis," an illness in which depression is the most prominent symptom; a person with a certain biogenetic and biochemical make-up may be exposed to certain stressful conditions which precipitate a "manic-depressive illness," the depressive phase of which is characterized by the symptom of depression.

In all three illnesses the person's lifelong inability to respond to his emotion of anger in a mature and effective manner is the most important cause for the development of the symptom of depression. To lose sight of this fact can cause treatment to be only partially effective. Drugs or electrotonic therapy can deal rather effectively with the worst of the melancholia episode; but unless the therapist is also able to help the woman deal in more mature ways with her anger, she is liable to have recurrences in her menopausal years.

On the other hand, when the therapist deals primarily with depression as a symptom of a lifelong failure to incorporate his emotion of anger, and secondarily uses antidepressant medication to lessen the depression and thus make cooperation in therapy possible, his chances of curing the patient permanently are much greater.

It is not hard to see how a person's inability to use his emotion of anger for the purpose of asserting and defending himself can make life increasingly miserable, if not unbearable. It is indeed depressing to be a doormat, to always give in to others, to be unable to make others mind your wishes and preferences, to be taken for granted, because of this emotionally crippling fear of anger.

God gave us the emotion of anger as one of the many instruments of our human nature that, when properly used under the guidance of the higher faculties, can make our lives more pleasant, successful and safe. Indeed, anger can be a tremendous stimulant in our overcoming great obstacles, in giving us endurance and determination. In some instances this emotion can be even a lifesaving factor.

This is illustrated dramatically by the prophet Isaiah's exclamation: "I have trodden the winepress alone. . . . I looked and there was none to help . . . none to uphold me . . . and my fury, it upheld me" (Isa. 63:3-5 author's paraphrase).

That the emotion of anger can be a lifesaving factor I experienced myself during my two years of imprisonment in the Nazi concentration camp of Buchenwald. Following my capture in the Pyrenées Mountains on the France-Spain border, endless interrogations about my participation in aiding Allied flyers escape from Europe, and stays in several French prisons, I was shipped with one thousand French prisoners to Buchenwald. Only six of us survived the long ordeal. Next to my faith in God, it was my constant anger at the Nazis for having deprived me of my liberty and their inhuman treatment of their prisoners that stimulated my determination to survive and to deny them the satisfaction of seeing me die. My anger stimulated my adrenal glands to provide me with energy to survive hard labor, a starvation diet and other hardships. Though I could never display my anger in any form, neither did I repress it. It was constantly directed by my reason which told me that to become outwardly angry at my captors would mean certain death. Prayer and anger allowed me to see the hour of liberation by General Patton and his Third Army. Nine hundred, ninety-four of the 1000 young Frenchmen in my transport from France to Buchenwald died, many of them as the result of their apathy and their lost *élan de vivre*. Without hope, afraid of their captors, they had lost the will to live. As a result they succumbed to minor illnesses and infectious diseases.

Ninety five percent of my patients recover from their depression when they learn to ask themselves, not, "Why am I so depressed?", but "What is annoying me; who is making me feel angry?" When they then identify the cause of their anger, and are helped to deal with that cause in ever more effective ways the depression lifts. One cannot be angry and feel depressed at the same time.

Chapter 7

Healing Emotional Afflictions

A long time ago the Lord told the prophet Ezekiel to say these words to the people: "I will give them new heart and put a new spirit within them; I will remove the stony heart from their bodies, and replace it with a natural heart, so that they will live according to my statutes, and observe and carry out my ordinances; thus they shall be my people and I will be their God" (Ezek. 11:19-20).

Those of us who have grown to chronological adulthood without a fully developed, well-balanced, and wholly integrated emotional life, often wonder *when* and how God will give us a new heart and spirit. Now that we know so much more about the preventable, man-made emotional disorders—the repressive and deprivation neuroses—that make our lives so unnecessarily difficult and sad, we have new hope that the time of fulfillment of God's promise to Ezekiel is near.

But when we think of *how* God will bring this about, we tend to be somewhat skeptical. The number of emotionally wounded and crippled people is so vast, and the number of qualified professionals so small in comparison, that short of a miracle we cannot imagine how all of us can receive the new hearts and spirits we so sorely need.

Yet, there is much that can be done with God's grace to help ourselves and one another. People need to know what neurotic conditions require professional help, and which neuroses are best treated by one kind of therapist, and which by another kind. People need to know in what areas of repression persons so afflicted can do a great deal for themselves, and in which they need help and advice from a professional. Furthermore, unaffirmed persons need to learn what they can do, and give up doing, in order to become most receptive to the unconditional love of others. And finally, all of us need and can learn how to pray with one another and thus to serve as the Lord's instruments for the healing power of His love.

I shall deal with all these topics to a reasonable extent and provide basic guidelines for further learning in some areas if this is needed and desired.

Q. Could you begin by explaining what unaffirmed persons can do to help themselves? You have said that their number is growing by leaps and bounds, and one sometimes wonders whether there are enough mature, affirmed persons left to make up for the parents who failed to give their children their psychic births. The unaffirmed people I have met often have an utter sense of helplessness because they believe there is nothing they themselves can do to facilitate this psychic birth,

this being opened to their own unique goodness by another person. They seem convinced that someone has to come along and use some method or technique of affirmation that will take away their feelings of loneliness, insecurity, inferiority, and so on. If this true, then I cannot see how all these unaffirmed people are going to receive the new heart the Lord has promised.

A. In the past several years I have realized that my choice of the word "affirmation" in the early sixties has been less enlightening than I expected it to be. In spite of defining it in books and lectures as an existential quality, as a way of *being*, too many people have interpreted it as something that is *done* for and unto others. Both the practical mentality of Western man and the distribution of poorly plagiarized books on affirmation seem to have contributed to this deplorable confusion. To provide some badly needed clarity I shall explain in a somewhat different terminology what has caused the unaffirmed person to become what he is, and how he can actively participate in his own healing, without being a self-affirmer.

The unaffirmed person did not grow to emotional maturity, because as a child he did not live in the orbit of persons who were living the affirming life.

He did not come to *feel* his own goodness, worth and loveableness because those significant persons in his life were not present to him with the full attention of their whole being.

Because others did not open him to his own unique goodness, he remained self-centered, afraid and unable to open himself to the world around him, to discover and experience the goodness of others, and of God.

As his "heart"—his humane emotions and intuitive mind—did not receive its proper nourishment, it remained undeveloped. Because of this he was forced to rely more and more on his "mind"—his thinking mind and utilitarian emotions—to pretend he was older than he felt, to act like others of his age, to fearfully protect himself from being hurt by other people, by not displeasing them, or to use his talents, or even other people, to make himself appear more important than he really felt.

As his "heart" atrophied and shrank, his "mind" grew excessively. Ever more fearful and withdrawn from people and the world, or driven to be busy and to achieve in restless pursuits, his capacity to be loved and to find joy in friendship grew smaller and smaller.

Becoming more weary and suspicious of the affirming *methods* applied by friends, counselors and therapists, which did nothing to make him feel loved for himself, he despaired even more of receiving what he *really* needed. He became more demanding of those who were able to satisfy his need, as his fear of being hurt again by pseudo-affirming or self-affirming others closed him off more to those who truly lived the affirming life.

This brief description of the fate of the unaffirmed person gives us all the clues as to what this person can *do* and *be* in order to become more receptive to those able and willing to love him unconditionally. In essence this requires that he must first *undo*, i.e., desist from, many of the activities of his "mind." Next, he must learn to *be* according to the needs of his "heart."

To make this possible he must first create and arrange

for conditions in his life that allow his undeveloped "heart" to do some growing. This requires knowledge of those conditions as well as determination, courage and perseverance to realize them. The unaffirmed person already possesses these qualities of courage and determination. He always employs them—to his own disadvantage—in ignoring slights and injustices and being nice to everyone, in making himself do what he does not feel like doing, and in putting up with the adult world in which he feels like a child. Thus, the unaffirmed person possesses ready-made qualities which, if redirected to the right goals, will enable him to live the first principles of the affirming life.

By doing this first in the world of things and beings that were created by God before He created man, he is not dependent on the adult world that inspires so much fear. He saves himself the discouragement and frustration of vainly trying to "earn" what can only be received as a gift. Thus the affectivity of his "heart" has a chance to develop to the point that eventually it can be open and receptive to the gift of himself by another.

Since the already affirmed person must do many of the same things to protect and maintain his *affectivity* against being stifled or destroyed by the *effectivity* surrounding and accosting him in his largely utilitarian milieu, I shall list the conditions to be created and preserved that make it possible to live the authentic human life—the affirming life.

Because one of the first principles of affirming living consists in being present to everything that is, with the full attention of one's entire being, the "mind" must be more silent than it usually is in our "rational" and rationalizing society. Normally, Western man meets every situation and person with an abundance of thoughts, judgments, opinions, comparisons, if not prejudgments and a know-it-all attitude. This he does for the purpose of being safe and prepared to protect himself from the unknown; to make the best use of certain circumstances; to take advantage of an opportunity; to gain information; to make a good impression on the other person; in short, to advance his utilitarian needs. Or he looks at the world without seeing it, because he is so busily engaged in the pursuit of happiness: "I have seen those trees, and flowers, and sunsets already before—I have more important things to do." His overdeveloped, overstimulated "mind" prevents his "heart" from being present with the awe and wonder of a child who sees a dandelion for the first time; from letting the unknown become part of him, to let the mystery of the unknown be and not demand it to be like the already known. His "mind" prevents his "heart" from being moved with love and joy and tenderness, from being authentically present to the other for the sake of the other.

The real meaning of *authentic presence* became even more clear to me when I was told of an Indian custom in the northwest region of our country. At a wake, which begins at dusk, no one speaks. The Indians enter the tent where the wake is held, shake hands in silence with the immediate relatives of the deceased, and sit all night in total silence around the body.[23]

The unaffirmed person, therefore, must dare to restrict the activity of his "mind" so his "heart" can be more open and sensitive. It takes courage to be open with the "heart," for one is more vulnerable when one relinquishes the protective workings of the "mind." For this reason the unaffirmed person must first apply these principles only to the world of animals, plants, minerals, to what we usually call *nature*. In that world he cannot be hurt as he has been hurt by the human beings who failed to be present to him. For the time being, while engaged in "natural or earthly contemplation" he must try not to "bother" with people, or at least to do so as infrequently as possible.

In order to reduce all unnecessary stimulation of his "mind," the unaffirmed person—like the affirmed person who must preserve his affectivity—must avoid all unnecessary distractions (the trivia offered by TV, radio, telephone, papers and magazines) and solve daily problems as soon as they arise. (This cuts down also on fear and anxiety.)

He must arrange as much as possible for greater quiet and more silence in his life. This he can do by avoiding the idle talk and chatter of others, and by refusing to participate in it himself. He must live more calmly and unhurriedly by setting priorities, avoiding overscheduling, limiting appointments, and refusing to give in to unreasonable demands on his time. A less demanding job in a more natural environment may have to be considered.

He must create opportunities and time for plentiful exposure to the immediate sources of nourishment of his "heart": the beauty of nature, pleasurable activities (fishing, playing, swimming, skiing and many others), the arts, philosophy, the Scriptures, meditation, divine contemplation—in short to all that is good, beautiful and true. Such exposures stimulate his emotions of love, joy and desire. He should avoid stimulation of more than one sense at a time, so he can give his full attention to what he senses via one sense. A good example of this is the avoidance of background music while eating, studying, sunbathing, etc.

By the same token he should avoid exposure to the bad, the ugly and false, so abundant in our secular, man-centered, utilitarian society that recognizes fewer and fewer absolute moral truths and God, and is bored by natural goodness and beauty.

The effect of all this is enhanced by doing what is possible to refine his external senses and his sense of imagination. Gourmet drinking and dining; attending symphonies, plays, ballets; good literature; visits to museums, and so on, all refine the senses. The imagination which has been most likely already overstimulated by fear and anxiety, must be helped to replace negative, paralyzing images with positive images which give new hope and courage and self-confidence.

For many persons it is not an easy matter to be converted from the abundance of distractions which they had sought for the very purpose of not having to be aware of themselves and conscious of their frustrated needs. When one has been led to believe that one is bad, unloveable, inferior, unwanted, etc., it is only natural to try and turn off these thoughts and feelings. Being always busy and on the go, constant exposure to TV and loud "music" or rock, drugs that cloud the mind, and many other devices that destroy peace and quiet, are the usual ways to close oneself off from what one fears to be, but actually is not.

It is often helpful to ease into the art of ever greater awareness of and receptive presence to all that is, including one's own self, by simply following one's normal breathing in an atmosphere of quiet, silence and relaxation; or simply listening to a symphony without trying to figure out who composed the music, or what instruments are being used, etc. One simply tries to be without doing. This process can be accelerated with the use of my self-help tapes available from the author.[24]

To the extent that he cannot avoid the company of other people, the unaffirmed person should gradually reduce and relinquish his ways of pleasing and impressing others for the purpose of "earning" their love. These other-pleasing ways and attempts to prove one's worth and loveableness are extensively described in *Healing the Unaffirmed* and should be studied carefully. Each person should list his own particular ways of compensating for not feeling loved and worthwhile, and then "work" at minimizing and abandoning these ways, while learning to be present to all that is in a new and healthy way. The more "honest" he can learn to be in recognizing and accepting his true emotions, and not give in to his fear of them, the more authentic will he be and the more meaningful the love and respect he will receive from others.

If the unaffirmed person is in the habit of putting other people down, however subtly, he should stop these and other ways of denying people, of not letting them be who they are. (Of course, if their ways are harmful or offensive to the unaffirmed person he should make this known in some way.) Putting other people down because they are different may give the unaffirmed person a momentary sense of being better, but it does not contribute in the least to the fulfillment of his need for authentic love. On the contrary, it does the very opposite. People do not like to be put down and do not love those who do this.

The unaffirmed person should make it as easy as possible for others to treat him better and with greater respect. This is done by letting them know what he likes, dislikes, feels, believes, expects, etc. He must go against his inclination to pretend that everything others say and do is agreeable with him, if in fact it is not.

Most unaffirmed persons, in their need for love, believe they must make every effort to love others and be loved by them. Rather he should direct all his efforts and energies at becoming comfortable with all of his emotions, not just that of love alone. He must learn to respond to his emotions and those of others without fear and in a variety of ways. This provides him with practical experiences and information about how his emotional responses can improve his life and relationships.

If the unaffirmed person is also an energy neurotic or workaholic, it is of great importance that he lives for an extended period of time in an undemanding, nonutilitarian milieu that permits him to be himself and live his life at his own pace.

Even before the unaffirmed person, who succeeds in following the foregoing advice, enters the orbit of others who live the affirming life, he will experience the following benefits of being wholly present to all that is.

In the growing communion—and decreased communication—with all that is good and beautiful and true in God's creation, he experiences greater calm and peace. His capacity to feel love and liking grows, and thus there is more joy that replaces the sadness of his erstwhile coping with the unaffirming adult world of people around him. Though avoiding those people more, he feels less lonely as he is more present to God's creation and feels its beauty and goodness as His gifts to him. These feelings are enhanced as he takes more time for meditating on the most consoling passages of the Scriptures and the words of unconditional love that Jesus spoke. In time there is an ever deeper sense of belonging and being loved for himself as his capacity for spiritual contemplation is facilitated by that for "earthly" contemplation. This is particularly true when the aforementioned willed techniques (of being quiet, being present to one's breathing, etc.) become "second nature" and thus create a *need* and *desire* to make the time available for being present to creation and the Creator.

His fears and anxiety decrease as he discovers that there is little to fear in nature, the arts and the teachings of God which, fortunately, are being taught and explained with ever less ambiguity and greater clarity. His trust grows, and so does his hope for becoming fully whole, and for sensing his own goodness and worth without doubts. As he turns to his emotions and feelings more, he allows himself to be guided more by them in such matters as eating only when he has an appetite (instead of a fixed number of times according to custom and convenience), and meeting friends and relatives more with what his "heart" tells him, rather than with the fear-inspiring thoughts of his "mind."

Of course, all this is only a beginning, an opening of the door from within by the unaffirmed person. But it is a most important beginning of a way of living that finds its completion in the other person or persons doing their part to open the door of his lonely, imprisoned self from the outside. Since the door had become heavier, and its hinges rustier than they once were in infancy and childhood—because significant others were unable or did not bother to open it during the growing years—those others must now give more of themselves to help the unaffirmed person open the door wide. This is definitely not a task for pseudo-affirming others who rely on techniques and methods of affirmation. Much less is it a task of self-affirming persons. In fact, the unaffirmed person must be protected and protect himself against these pseudo-affirming and self-affirming persons who only close doors, and never open them so the unaffirmed person can be set free from his prison of loneliness.

But when the unaffirmed person, who as the result of creating for himself the conditions I have described, is ready to live with a reasonable degree of openness in the orbit of the person who truly lives the affirming life, the process of becoming who he is supposed to be is ready to be completed.

Not too long ago, on one of my lecture tours I met a Protestant minister who had suffered for years from a deep depression that no drugs or shock treatment had been able to alleviate. After reading *Born Only Once* he had decided to concentrate on doing nothing but simply being present to what he called all the little things around him. This he did in a spirit of praise and gratitude to God who had created those little things for his happiness. Proceeding from inanimate objects to flowers, pets and little children, he gradually lost his loneliness, fears and depression. The children especially made him feel that he belonged and that he was loved by them and God. From there it was only a small step to feel at ease and happy with the people who made up his parish and with his work.

This account by the healed minister emphasizes the need to follow my instructions regarding affirming living in a spirit of praise and gratitude to God. Thus the Christian unaffirmed person, in learning to live the affirming life, accelerates the process by giving praise and thanks to God every time he is present to what He has created: the grass, weeds, pebbles, trees, flowers, sunshine, rain and all else. The same is true for the man-made objects in his life, for they also are presents to him from God who used his fellow human beings in their construction: the bed, pillow, car, house, window, utensils, food, light bulbs, vacuum cleaner, and on and on.

"Lord, I praise and thank you for the house that protects me from the elements; I praise and thank you for the water from the faucet that I use for so many purposes; I thank and praise you for the electricity that operates the toaster, the washing machine, etc." These simple, quiet, oft repeated observations of the things we usually take for granted in a spirit of thanks and praise is a most effective antidote to the counter-productive, utilitarian ways of looking at things.

It is almost second nature for many people to focus on what is imperfect, missing, inadequate, and bad in the *present* with feelings of discontent and frustration. Others focus with feelings of worry and anxiety on what may happen in the *future*, on the unknown, possible sickness, lack of work and money, death, etc. Others focus with feelings of regret and bitterness on mistakes, setbacks, painful memories, frustrations of the *past*. To make the switch from this addictive habit of looking only at the negative to being present to the world around us in praise and gratitude to God can be difficult. This is particularly true for persons whose fear or mistrust of God has led them to believe that everything is up to their own efforts. Yet nothing is impossible, and once they follow the above advice, the effects become quickly noticeable in terms of growing inner peace and "passive" energy, and a host of other benefits. In time, when one has matured more, one will also be able to give praise and thanks to God for permitting misfortune, pain and sufferings, in the certain faith that He will use them to bring about a greater good.

Q. Should a person have any special knowledge of what to be and do for the unaffirmed person he wants to help become himself?

A. No and yes. If that person is already living the affirmed life fully, he just "knows" how to let the other be, and allow him to become himself at his own pace and in his own way. By being present to him with his "heart," and feeling comfortable with his feelings of love and compassion, and not embarrassed to "reveal" these feelings naturally and spontaneously, but refraining from those expressions that do not constitute a good for the unaffirmed person, the unaffirmed person will *feel* the goodness, beauty, and worth of his own person.

For him this "revelation" is life-giving, creative, strengthening, healing. It lays the psychological foundation for what can be perfected only by the Holy Spirit when a person willingly and freely, and under the proper circumstances and conditions, opens himself to this Spirit.

The fruit of the Holy Spirit is: love, joy, peace, patience, kindness, generosity, faithfulness, gentleness and self-control. We become recipients of this fruit when other persons use His gifts—faith, knowledge, wisdom, prophecy, tongues, interpretation, miracles, healing, discernment of spirits for our benefit, not for their own benefit.[25]

This is precisely what the person who lives the affirming life does. He shares what he has received as a gift from others, with those not yet gifted, and thus gives them the gift of themselves and thereby joy, peace, and love. When these natural gifts of the person who lives the affirming life are complemented by the gifts of the Holy Spirit, the fruit of the Holy Spirit complements the natural effects of his affirming life in the not-yet-affirmed persons.

Though the Spirit blows where He wills, in the natural course of events the Spirit works through others. He seems to prefer human beings to be His co-creators, co-affirmers, co-healers. It is an "unbeatable" combination, the Holy Spirit and man cooperating in bringing life, strength and healing to mankind. Obviously, this truth imposes a serious obligation on every human being to live the affirming life, and thus to be an authentic "revealer" or "strengthener" of his fellow-man. He cannot simply leave it up to God or to the other person himself to become what he is meant to be. He is needed as a co-creator!

The foregoing explains why it was proper for me to

reply *no* to the question as to whether a person requires special knowledge about what to be and do for the unaffirmed person. But because there are so many pseudo-affirming persons who with their writings and practices have caused so much confusion—and harm—I had to answer also *yes*.

These pseudo-affirming persons, who use the word "affirmation" so freely, and are so busy "affirming" others with their *techniques of doing*, do not know what the person who lives the affirming life knows. In fact, the pseudo-affirming person will have no idea that I have omitted something very important in what I have just described as "life-giving, creative, strengthening, healing, revelation." Only the person who lives the affirming life knows that my comparison between his gifts and those of the Holy Spirit was not as complete and explicit as it should be.

It is this one aspect, which I purposely omitted, which distinguishes the person who leads the authentic affirming life from the one who does not and pushes the "button of affirmation" in counseling; who devises new affirmation techniques for group encounters; who stresses emotions and feelings at the expense of moral truths; who makes a living turning out self-help books and offering pop-psychology courses which do not consider, or are ignorant of, the intellectual and spiritual needs of man. The pseudo-affirmers, or worse, the self-affirmers, engaged in counseling and related fields, are recognizable by the fact that they do not lead the affirming life themselves. This is not always easy to ascertain, for many pseudo-affirmers are of good will, sincere in wanting to help others, and are tireless in doing what they can, even to the point of exhausting themselves and becoming sick.

But it is precisely because they *do* (and not because they *are*) that their services and help to unaffirmed people must be labeled pseudo-affirming. Frequently, these same people are also the willing supporters of the new educational approaches which are devastating in so many ways to the unaffirmed children in our society. They copy these new developments with great enthusiasm and are blissfully unaware of how they defeat their own, already inadequate, efforts to help others grow and become themselves. (See next chapter.)

Q. What is it that you have purposefully omitted, and which should be an essential aspect of my affirming living if the unaffirmed person is to benefit fully from living in my orbit?

A. Perhaps I should have anticipated that in our feeling-dominated times many people would ignore what we described explicitly in our books as being a fundamental need for the unaffirmed person.[26] He needs not only emotional strengthening, but also intellectual strengthening. He needs not only to *feel* the truth that he is loveable and good, but also to *know how to live the truth*, how to live according to the laws of his nature and those of the One who created his nature. Without knowledge of these laws he is unable to establish order in his life and to avoid whatever is detrimental to his relationship with God and his fellow human beings.

This need is forgotten, if it ever was understood, by the many who are anxious to affirm others but are not yet affirmed themselves. Sure, they often, as part of their "doing-affirmation," give abundant advice and a variety of "musts" and "should nots" to the unaffirmed person, but frequently this advice is of a subjective and feeling nature. By this I mean, they tell him what they feel he should do, what they feel is right for him. This kind of "teaching" predominates in our times, in which powerful voices are heard in opposition to "indoctrination of absolute values," to the existence of objective truths, and to God himself.

But this kind of "knowledge," this clarification of moral values on the basis of emotional reactions, is *not* what the unaffirmed person needs. He needs neither emotional junk food, nor intellectual half-truths and falsehoods. Just as he remains emotionally a child when pseudo-affirmers feed him emotional junk food, so does he slowly suffocate when they expose him to the indoctrination of their own value clarifications, or of their psycho-theological quicksand.[27]

Q. Where do unaffirmed children and adults, once their emotional growth has advanced sufficiently, find the necessary knowledge to establish order in their lives, to live a virtuous life that brings them reasonable happiness in this world, and to enjoy lasting happiness in the after life?

A. I believe everyone must find the answer to this question for himself. However, he will have a better chance to succeed when he is able to recognize the educational pitfalls of present day public and private schools, seminaries and convents, as well as the shortcomings of modern innovations in mainline churches, newly arising religious cults, and self-help movements.

With the appearance of new and often better pedagogical approaches in education and religion, content has frequently been watered down, and in some cases the baby (content) has been thrown out together with the bath water (process). But it is exactly the long-established truths of the past that have not always been conserved by the change-loving liberals, which constitute the much needed food of intellectual strengthening. The fact that in the past these truths were too often presented in an authoritarian manner, which tolerated no questioning and requests for clarification, does not mean that those truths have been proven false. Too often, the liberals' justified rebellion against immature, dictatorial, self-seeking authority of the past has aimed at abolishing authority and replacing it with government by consensus. Their failure to work at helping authority to become mature, and govern as affirmed and affirming individuals, has harmed the unaffirmed person greatly. Mature, affirmed persons in authority are an indispensable source of much needed strength and growth for their subjects.

Because of their emotional uncertainty in living, unaffirmed persons have a greater than average need to know the fundamental rules of living. The historical, philosophical and religious truths, as taught for example by the magisterium of the Catholic Church and the liberal arts colleges, have always been our primary sources of knowledge. Regrettably, the former has somewhat suffered of late in her credibility, while the latter have dwindled in number throughout the Western world.

Unaffirmed persons are not strengthened by a utilitarian education that prepares them for a job, even when this education is presented in a socio-psycho-therapeutic atmosphere aimed at meeting the emotional needs of the students. It is not fair to expect teachers to make up for the failures of unaffirmed and unaffirming parents, and to bring order in the emotionally disordered lives of their students, while at the same time having to tend to their duty of teaching them something more than trivia. But do they have a choice?

Education that is worthy of the name aims at the development of the student's capacity to think, reason, form opinions and judgments. Internal emotional underdevelopment, frustration and turmoil seriously interferes with his responsiveness. Under these disabling and frustrating conditions all that can be done is to *train* him to act in the earnest and least demanding way. Usually this amounts to training him to hold a job that requires little more than operating certain machines and performing routine tasks.

I hope these brief reflections will stimulate a rethinking on the part of parents and teachers about young people's emotional and educational needs.

Q. Is it correct to summarize your teachings on affirming living—in the context of the needs of unaffirmed persons—by saying that this consists of being present with the full attention of one's whole being—with "heart" and "mind," and of teaching intellectual and spiritual truths?

A. Yes, it is. But I want to add something regarding the second part of your summary. It is not only necessary for the affirmed person to *know* those truths and to be *willing* to teach them. He also must have the *ability* to present them *at the right time* to a particular unaffirmed person, and *in the right ways*, ways that are adjusted and suited to that person's emotional needs and degree of strength at any given time of his growth.

This presentation also includes the capacity to correct,

to admonish, to use, if need be, strong language that leaves no doubt as to the gravity of the matter at hand. It recognizes and respects the unaffirmed person's needs, and "where he is, and comes from," but does not hesitate to offer truths in such a manner that he is open to them and capable of receiving and responding to them.

This naturally takes great sensitivity and experience, as well as the other qualities that are the characteristics of the already affirmed person. But it is here that the pseudo-affirming and self-affirming persons fail, even when they possess adequate knowledge of established truths. Their affirmation techniques usually are practiced in an atmosphere of permissiveness and "sensitivity" directed at not "hurting anyone's feelings."

All I have presented here concerning the affirming life is most clearly illustrated in the life of the first affirmer of man, Jesus Christ. Jesus came to earth to *preach* the good news, and to *live* the good news. Jesus strengthened man's need to know truths by *preaching* the good news, since then preserved in the Scriptures. He presented these truths either directly and explicitly, or in parables, or in simple, almost incidental ways, but these were always adjusted to the level of development of the persons in His audience. He never compromised on these truths. He did not hesitate to use strong language, even though it would be sure to hurt the listeners' feelings: "Woe to you scribes and Pharisees, you frauds! . . . blind guides. . . . Blind fools. . ." (Matt. 23:13-17).

Jesus *lived* the good news in His relationship with His apostles and the women with whom He shared much of His private life. Here He did His real, most effective teaching of people's loveableness in the eyes and heart of

God. This teaching of the affirming life by Jesus was not done as I had to do it here, in words and laying down of principles, and pointing out pitfalls, and so on. He taught it in His way of being. To live the truth is always the most effective way of teaching the truth. Unfortunately, this way of teaching can be made available only to a limited number of persons. The multitudes must be satisfied with articles and books describing the truths lived by a certain person among his family, students, friends and associates. These fortunate few then have the task of promulgating those truths in their turn: first of all in living them, and secondarily, through oral teachings.

And so it was with the apostles whom Jesus chose to be His co-affirmers, co-creators of other people. For three years Jesus compassionately revealed to them their own goodness in His intimate, authentic presence to them, until they in turn were ready, following their conversion, to *strengthen their brothers* (Luke 22:32). The New Testament is replete with examples of how Jesus' teachings of truths were often preceded by His special ways of opening a person's heart with His sensitive, compassionate presence. Jesus knew what too often we forget or never have known, that the way to convince another person of a truth is not so much by logical arguments, but via the "heart" ("and the Lord opened her [Lydia's] heart to accept what Paul was saying" [Acts 16:14]).

When Jesus, or we, are authentically present to another person, and he as a result *feels* his own hidden goodness, he is so moved with gratitude that he is open to whatever other good Jesus, or we, have to offer him. ("Saul, Saul, why do you persecute me? It is hard for you to kick against the goad" [Acts 26:14]—and immediately

Paul was converted).

When our presence is always authentic and we teach the truth in the right way, at the right time, the other person becomes stronger and will possess himself in peace and joy, capable of revealing to others the truth of their goodness and those of God and His creation. Under those circumstances one does not have to be afraid to "hurt a person's feelings" with the truth. That person's strength will not be shattered, because he *knows* and *feels* secure in the authentic presence of another.

This is dramatically demonstrated by Jesus—who always affirmed, never denied, not even in His strongest denunciations—in His encounter with Peter. After nearly three years of revealing to Peter his unique goodness, and even his hidden strength of being a rock (Matt. 16:18), Jesus teaches Peter a supernatural truth at the very moment when Peter shows his deep love of Jesus by declaring that he wants Jesus to be spared from suffering and death. At that moment "Jesus turned on Peter and said, 'Get out of my sight, you satan! You are trying to make me trip and fall. You are not judging by God's standards but by man's" (Matt. 16:23).

These are unkind, harsh, unchristian words to persons who are not familiar with the meaning of the affirming life. To them these words are spoken by the man Jesus because He is also God, and therefore can permit himself an exception to the rule of always being gentle. Just as they tend to believe that as God, Jesus had the right to deviate from His teaching of "turning the other cheek," when He became so angry that He fashioned a whip and used it on the moneychangers in the temple.

Those familiar with the meaning of the affirming life, and living it themselves, understand that these were the perfect affirming words spoken by Jesus. Perfect, because they were said to Peter who had grown strong enough not to be shattered by "hurt feelings," and to be capable of learning the gravity of a particular supernatural truth.

This particular passage is an excellent demonstration of the truth that *no authentic teaching is possible by a pseudo-affirmer, much less by a self-affirmer.* As he does not strengthen others with his techniques and methods of affirmation, they remain fragile and will be easily hurt when told even an authentic truth. The pseudo-affirming atmosphere of being "nice," and saying the right things, of being tolerant and permissive, reveals the lack of authenticity of the person claiming to "practice affirmation." By just being with such a person for a while, one can sense the lack of authentic presence and authentic teaching. Such presence and teaching always radiate serenity, calm and peace.

I once was invited to give a series of lectures by a sister in charge of a diocesan formation center. She had heard me lecture for a period of five days and had become so enthusiastic with the concept of affirmation that she began to practice it right away in her sincere desire to help others grow. It was two years later before I was able to respond to her invitation to lecture in her diocese. Sad to say, her efforts proved to be nothing but pseudo-affirming practices. She had organized numerous groups and was involved in all kinds of organizations where she was busy "affirming" the people and teaching them to affirm others. In the hours she spent with me, introducing me, chauffeuring me to different meeting halls, taking me out to dinner, I never felt a moment of peace. With all her talk about affirmation, I never felt her being present to me. On the contrary, I almost felt denied, for I had little chance to be myself, except during the hours of lecturing and responding to questions and comments of the audience.

Even worse is the feeling one experiences when meeting a self-affirming person who claims to be engaged in affirmation therapy. Some of these persons direct centers that are designated as such and write affirmation books. They are more subtle in their deceit, for they are more clever, if not masters, in pretending that their actions stem from compassion. It may take longer to sense their self-seeking and striving for power, but it can never remain hidden indefinitely.

Q. Can self-affirming people be healed, or help themselves?

A. If one were to approach them with the advice that they need help with their underdeveloped emotional life, they most likely would not know what you are talking about and tell you to mind your own business. Or, they might tell you it is your problem that you feel unloved by them, even though your love for them is real. They will continue living their lives in the only way they know—striving for fame, power, influence, riches, sexual love—and, if you are not careful, they will not hesitate to manipulate you in the process.

Self-affirmation may be compared to a cancer. Its cells feed on the surrounding healthy cells, and thus destroy them in the process. The cancer cells grow and multiply at a faster rate than normal cells, invade healthy tissues mercilessly and resist attempts to destroy and eradicate them. More often than not, the self-affirming cancer cells destroy the body in which they grow and thus ultimately also themselves.

It is only if and when at last self-affirming persons discover that there is nothing but a void at the top of the ladder they have so strenuously climbed, that they may become open to their need for help, provided their depression does not become so severe as to precipitate suicide. But it is at that point that the frustrated self-affirming person can help himself by learning to live the affirming life, though by that time he may have his more advanced age against him.

Q. What can psychiatrists do for the more severely disabled deprivation neurotic, especially when he is deeply depressed and wishes to be dead?

A. The answer to your question is covered extensively in the book, *Healing the Unaffirmed*. There is no need to duplicate this here as the book is readily available from the publisher and bookstores.

We must end here the discussion of the healing of unaffirmed persons in order to have more time to describe that of other emotionally afflicted people.

Q. Dr. Baars, earlier you remarked that repressive neurotics should be treated by professionals. Does this mean that you are not going to tell us anything about the kind of therapy you think is best for these neurotics? In my opinion it would be helpful for the nonprofessionals to know a little about this, so parents, teachers, clergy and others will know to whom to refer the different kinds of repressive neurotics.

A. The therapies for repressive neurotics are described in depth in *Healing for Neurotics*. Both professionals and nonprofessionals will find in this book a presentation of the particular form of therapy my colleague, Dr. Anna Terruwe, and I employ in treating those persons who suffer with obsessive-compulsive neuroses. It is written in a style that is understandable to the nonprofessional who likes to expand his knowledge of these matters for whatever reason. At the same time it gives the professional person sufficient data for adjusting his present therapies for repressive neurotics.

What nonprofessionals should know about the treatment of repressive neuroses is that the hysterical neurotic, in my opinion, is best served by the psychoanalyst. His probing approach aims at bringing the repressed emotion into consciousness. This is necessary because the emotion has been placed beyond the guidance by reason, and thus beyond control of the will. The hysterical neurotic as a rule is completely unaware of the fact that he has repressed a certain emotion or feeling, and of how this is active in his unconscious and causes the hysterical symptoms that are obvious to everyone save the patient himself. The analyst, therefore, uses all the customary techniques to uncover the repressed emotion, so that the patient will become aware of it, and literally sense it to be alive within him. (The mere knowledge on his part that he is likely to harbor a hidden emotion is not enough by itself.) At that point the analyst must aid the patient in finding the proper means of responding to the emotion in a rational manner. As soon as that happens the hysterical symptom will no longer serve any useful function and it will disappear.

This does not mean that the successful resolution of a hysterical symptom (e.g., blindness, paralysis, or the like) guarantees there will be no recurrence. In fact, recurrences are likely because it is very difficult to effect such a change in the personality structure of the hysterical neurotic, that he will never again resort to repression as a way of dealing with certain emotional stress. As I mentioned before, hysterical neurotics are usually of low normal, or below normal intelligence, and deficient in introspective power. For these reasons they do not lend themselves to fundamental personality modifications necessary to prevent future recurrences of hysterical symptoms.

Therefore, the best thing nonprofessionals can do for persons with such symptoms as I described earlier is to refer them to a psychoanalyst.

The same is not true when it comes to advising persons with an obsessive-compulsive neurosis. These persons should not be referred to psychoanalysts, but to those psychiatrists who are in agreement that it is not the superego, but rather an emotion of the utility appetite—fear or/and energy—which is responsible for the neurotic repression. This distinction makes a fundamental difference in the therapy of obsessive-compulsive neurotics. These persons are intellectually so aware of the life they lead, so busily occupied with their own emotional experiences, and so intensely concerned with either controlling their emotional stirrings or avoiding whatever might stimulate feared emotions, that the complete unawareness and absolute autonomy of their symptoms, so typical in hysterical neurotics, is an impossibility.

The essential feature of an obsessive-compulsive neurosis is the forceful repression of an emotion by another emotion—fear or/and energy—stimulated as they are by a misinformed intellect. From a therapeutic point of view, therefore, it does not make sense deliberately, through analytic probing, to bring more repressed material into the patient's consciousness. If one were to do this without simultaneously alleviating the repressing emotion(s), one would merely intensify the repressive process and make the illness worse.

In these persons the therapy must be directed first of all at reducing the repressing emotions to a more normal intensity, namely, diminishing the fear or curtailing the excessive energy. By doing this the repression will lose its force and the repressed emotions will gradually emerge by themselves into consciousness, where they can find adequate release under normal rational control.

I have decided that a full discussion of this therapeutic process as far as sexual repression is concerned cannot be included in this book. Its closely associated moral aspects make the resolving of repressed sexual feelings a most delicate procedure. Its presentation would require a lengthier and more scholarly discussion than is possible in the scope of this book. However, a full exposé of this topic will be included in *Healing for Neurotics*, especially the effect of neurotic repression on the freedom of the will.

I want to refer professionals and persons actively engaged in the ministry of inner healing to that book. It will give theologians, spiritual directors, ministers, and qualified religious men and women in pastoral work a thorough understanding of the pertinent psychological and psychiatric aspects of the therapy of obsessive-compulsive neurotics, which will enable them to provide the psychiatrist and patient with sound advice concerning the moral aspects of the patient's behavior during therapy.

Christians suffering from scrupulosity and other forms

of obsessive-compulsive neurosis can rest assured that our particular interpretation of the repressive process, and our principles of its therapeutic resolution, are morally responsible and psychiatrically effective. Whether the same is true for the therapy of the Freudian psychoanalyst and the behavioral psychologist is something that cannot be claimed categorically. I assume that the individual Christian analyst or behaviorist always takes pains to refrain from giving advice that is in conflict with the moral laws. However, most Christian readers familiar with the extremely liberal positions in matters of sexual behavior advocated by "mental health" experts and certain theologians in our day will realize the need for a careful investigation of the therapist.

Q. I am somewhat disappointed that you cannot discuss here the therapy of sexual repression because of its delicate nature. Does the same hold true for the treatment of the repression of anger?

A. No. I shall be happy to outline the salient points in the treatment of persons who have repressed their angry feelings. By my doing this you will also learn the essential approach in the treatment of sexual repression. But for the answers to the questions that may form in your mind about the moral aspects of teaching a person to stop repressing his sexual feelings, you will have to turn to *Healing for Neurotics*.

The person who from early life was made to repress his feelings of anger must learn first of all to rid himself from the notion that it is bad for him to *feel* this emotion. If moral teachings about the actual or potential sinfulness of anger were the reason that the person as a child became fearful of anger, or driven to overcome his angry feelings, then these teachings must be ignored. This usually requires that the person understands the goodness of anger as an emotional tool given to us by God as an intrinsic part of our human nature for a positive purpose. He should have a good grasp of all I have written here about man's emotional life, and about anger in particular. Then without condemning or blaming his religious beliefs or religion itself, he must substitute: "I may feel angry" for "I must never feel angry" or "I'm afraid to be angry." This is an internal process of continued and repeated assurance that there is nothing to be afraid of, and that it is all right, in fact, desirable and necessary, to feel anger whenever one is exposed to situations that provoke this emotion. This process can be accelerated with the use of self-help tapes available from the author.

This process of inward reassurance is aimed at mortifying one's irrational fear of anger or one's being emotionally driven to overcome it. It does not call for any external action by the person. In fact, he should avoid doing or saying anything for the purpose of expressing his anger, until he *feels* quite comfortable and at ease whenever he feels angry, irritated, annoyed, mad, etc.

As this process may well take weeks or months, it is important that one is patient and does not attempt to speed up the recovery process, by expressing one's anger or asserting oneself prematurely (i.e., before all vestiges of fear or energy or feelings of guilt in response to feeling anger have disappeared). The advice often given to the effect that "You are much too passive and nonassertive; I want you to start growing up and get mad when people step on you," should be ignored. To force oneself to do this, in order to please the person who gave that advice, only aggravates the neurotic process.

Sometimes people have repressed their angry feelings so deeply for so many, many years that they have to start making a special effort to identify their feelings of irritation or anger. They may have to be like Sherlock Holmes for a while, looking for clues as to what they may be feeling, or even asking themselves, "Am I feeling anything at all? I *know* so-and-so didn't treat me right, but what do I *feel*?" Some have become masters at short-circuiting their feelings of irritation by "thinking them away" at the very first stirrings. For instance, as soon as they begin to feel irritated when someone lights up a cigarette in a nonsmoking area, they will think of an excuse for that person's behavior (e.g., "He probably didn't see the sign, or he really needs it; besides it won't be long before he puts it out; I'd probably do the same thing if I were he," etc.). These are all rationalizations aimed at not having to admit to one's feelings of annoyance or anger.

Or they may have reinforced their repression of anger by always saying, "I shouldn't feel angry at such a small and insignificant thing; nobody else gets angry at such little things." Those persons must learn to accept and own every emotion whenever it is felt, without criticizing themselves for feeling it. It makes no sense at all to say, "I should not feel this or that," or to others, "*You* shouldn't feel this way or that."

Even if you were the only person in the world to feel irritated, when someone, let us say, uses the word "please" (to give a ridiculous example), neither you nor anyone else can criticize you for feeling that way. It may be very odd and inexplainable, but the word "please" happens to stimulate in you the feeling of irritation. It may be necessary and advisable to find out *why* you feel that way, but it should not be done because you or others think, "You shouldn't feel that way." You *feel* it, and you *may* feel it. Then, when you accept that feeling of anger, you are free to do with it, and with the cause of the feeling, whatever you want. This you cannot do, however, if you respond with fear or energy; these emotions force you to repress the angry feelings and deprive you of the opportunity to deal with the cause of the feeling in a rational and sensible manner.

During this period of spotting, recognizing, accepting, and telling yourself over and over that it is all right to feel angry, and that you are grateful for feeling more and more comfortable with that feeling; of petitioning and thanking God for helping you to recognize His goodness also in your feeling anger—and all other emotions—practice *calling a spade a spade*. By this I mean, instead of using such expressions as "I am so upset," or "so hurt," say "I am so angry," or "mad." The use of the term "hurt" is particularly disabling and an obstacle to becoming emotionally aroused toward being capable of dealing effectively with the cause of the anger. Whether the user realizes it or not, the word "hurt" conjures up a visual image of being wounded, incapacitated, lying prostrate and helpless on the ground, waiting for the ambulance to come and the doctor to take care of him. He can't help himself; he is hurt and helpless.

In sharp contrast is the effect of the use of the word "angry" or "mad." The person who proclaims that he is angry visualizes himself standing up, ready to fight, if necessary, to protect himself and others. He is *not* helpless, but stimulated to do what is necessary.

The foregoing is not intended to mean that "hurt" is synonymous with "anger." The noun "hurt" indicates an "injury—blow or insult—that causes bodily or mental pain."[28] This mental pain is something like the feeling of grief, sorrow, sadness. However, when the hurt person reflects on the cause of the injury, he may well feel anger when, for instance, he realizes that someone he thought to be his good friend has offended him.

Neurotics often skip this reflective process because they are not comfortable with their angry feelings. They remain "stuck" in the "hurt" phase. Because the humane emotions as such—grief, sadness—do not directly stimulate a person to move or act—only *to be moved*—he remains passive. Only when sadness is followed by the utilitarian emotion of anger do the adrenal glands secrete the necessary amount of adrenaline to move him to defend himself.

In a mature, fully integrated person these two emotions—one humane, the other utilitarian—occur virtually simultaneously. We only have to look at Jesus to realize how true this is. When the Pharisees were watching Jesus to see whether He would cure a man with a withered arm on the Sabbath, Jesus asked them: "Is it permitted to do good or to do evil on the Sabbath, to save life or to kill?" When the Pharisees did not answer Him, Jesus began "looking round at them with anger and sorrow at their obstinate stupidity," and He went ahead and restored the arm (Mark 3:1-6, NEB). The New American Bible reveals even more clearly the succession of the emotions felt by Jesus: "He looked around at them with anger, for he was deeply grieved that they had closed their minds against him."

Once the person has been desensitized against

repressing his anger by means of fear or energy, and is reasonably comfortable when his anger is aroused, *then and only then* is he ready to experiment with actions aimed at dealing with the source of his anger.

Being inexperienced he must expect to make mistakes and be willing to learn from them. He must not demand instant perfection on the road toward learning mature, reasonable, sensible and, above all, *effective* responses to anger-provoking situations and people. He is to remember that it normally takes the first eighteen years of a person's life to learn what responses to feeling angry are the best in this or that situation, depending on who or what is involved, and what is at stake.

Not that it will take the adult as long a period, but quick, spontaneous, direct responses take some time to learn. As he is already physically and intellectually grown up, he will learn much quicker than the still-growing child and adolescent, provided, of course, he has the courage to "live dangerously," to take risks.

Q. What about the person who has repressed his angry feelings, not because of incorrect or untimely teachings, but because he was often traumatized by the irrational, angry outbursts of his parents, and their undeserved beatings and punishments?

A. Here the situation is a little different. Some of these persons decide at an early age never to hurt others as they have been hurt by their parents, and learn to *suppress* their angry feelings. They are aware of the anger they feel but will not express it, in the belief that anger is always and solely associated with harming others. They must be taught that there are many other ways of responding to their angry feelings, ways that are not harmful, socially acceptable, and above all Christian, in the sense that they can provide the offending person with opportunities to treat them better in the future.

If they hold their anger inside, they not only will suffer in time the effects of growing resentments, but also deprive the anger-provoking person of learning that he has offended or treated them unjustly. They deprive that person of the opportunity to make amends, apologize or mend his ways and treat others in a more Christian and loving way in the future.

A brief explanation of the difference between "repression" and "suppression" will make it clear why it is easier for persons who have suppressed their anger to be healed, than for those who have repressed it. Repression is a *subconscious* process and the person is often not aware of what is going on regarding his feeling of anger.

Suppression is a *conscious* process. The person knows that he feels anger but decides, for the wrong reasons, not to express it. For example, he may believe that it is always immature to show anger, or that anger never gets you anywhere. This belief prevents his anger from being guided by reason (e.g., "In this particular situation it would be stupid to become angry, because my boss is in such a bad mood that he'd fire me on the spot. I'll wait for another opportunity to deal with the cause of my anger"). However, because the *suppressing* person knows what he does, he is often helped more readily than the *repressing* person who must learn first to mortify his repressing feeling of fear and/or energy.

Q. Does the foregoing also apply to unaffirmed people who refrain from becoming angry?
A. No. The situation is different with them. You know

already that unaffirmed people usually do not deal with their assertive feelings as they should, because they consider the showing of their anger as a threat to their intense need to be loved. These persons must be helped in a way that differs from that for repressive neurotics. Of course, if a person has both types of neuroses, both treatments must and can be offered simultaneously.

Let me describe the principles of helping an unaffirmed person to use his feelings of anger to his advantage.

"Pure" unaffirmed people are not afraid of their emotions. They were never made to repress them. If they do not "express" certain feelings, like hate and anger, it is because they are afraid this would "turn off" other people whose love they like to receive or fear to lose. Once they lose this fear, they begin to make better use of their feelings of anger. In other words, nothing special has to be done to help the unaffirmed person with his feeling of anger. All that is needed is that he receives authentic affirmation. This will allow the heart of his entire emotional life to grow to the level of the adult.

While this growth takes place, the person will benefit from learning more about the function and purpose of anger as an emotion, and how its discreet "handling" can, in fact, speed up the process of feeling secure with others. He certainly should learn that anger does not need to be expressed as anger, as angry, heated words or violent action. In fact, in the truly adult world there are many better ways of reacting to one's angry feelings, ways that hold the promise of greater effectiveness in dealing with the *cause* of one's angry feelings:

A polite remark that one does not care to be treated in a certain way; a quiet hint that one expects an apology for having been offended; a question as to why the other acted as he did even though he knew it would cause one to feel angry; a firm communication that one does not expect to be treated the same way ever again; an announcement that one will take up the anger-producing situation at a more suitable time (to regain one's composure or not to involve others, etc.).

These and many, many other reactions are usually much more effective than the reactions uppermost in the minds of many in association with "expressing one's anger," or "getting angry": yelling, cursing, hitting, physical abuse, breaking things. For this reason I prefer to speak of "responding to one's feeling of anger" instead of "expressing one's anger." In the truly adult person, anger is rarely expressed as the fore-mentioned extremes of anger, but as reasonable responses dealing as directly and effectively as possible with the anger-provoking person and his words or actions.

If an unaffirmed person has never learned to do this, he must start later in life, be patient with himself, and allow himself sufficient time to become more adept and effective in a process that requires multiple and varied experiences in different situations and with different people. He will discover that the mature ways of dealing with his anger are more pleasing to others than his accommodating, "nice" ways, and much more likely to lead to friendships, love and respect.

Let me add some more pointers to facilitate the process of integrating the feeling of anger in your total personality.

You will know when the process is more or less complete when you have no need any more to speak of "handling your anger" or "dealing with your anger." After all, we do not apply the same terms to our legs and fingers, the other tools God has given us as part of our nature. Once we have learned to use them and no longer stumble and fall, or clumsily drop things from our hands, we use them automatically. If we were to start "dealing with them" and give particular attention to the way we put one foot in front of the other, we would stumble and fall, because this interferes with the natural process of walking. That is our goal in integrating our angry feelings, and all our emotions: to feel and respond to them in a natural, appropriate and spontaneous manner.

You will recall that I said earlier that in the matter of emotions, "It is all or nothing," (i.e., when you repress one emotion, the others will suffer the same fate—though to a lesser degree).

Therefore, the person who has always repressed or suppressed anger must now also aid his other emotions to become more a part of him. For a while he must make it a point to be more sensitive to his feelings of *love* of the beauty of nature, of *desire* to be in the company of a good friend, of *joy* when listening to soul-stirring music, of *compassion* when visiting a sick relative in the hospital, of *kindness* for a little child, of *gentleness* with a beggar, of *affection* with spouse and children, of *sadness* when hearing bad news, and so on.

And when even the bodily feelings have suffered in the years of repression, then he must also gradually cultivate his awareness of and responsiveness to his bodily sensations, in a spirit of appreciation and gratitude to God for having provided him with taste buds, sense of smell, tactile sense organs, and the like. Those senses, too, contribute to his joy of life provided those sense organs are adequately developed and are gratified insofar as this is reasonable according to the laws of nature and God.

As long as there is too much *talk* about emotions and feelings, there is not yet enough *experiencing* of them comfortably and spontaneously. It indicates that the person who "talks" emotions still has a way to go to feel them and make them his own. This is also true for those who use the word "affirmation" all the time, whether in conversation, relating to others, training or treatment groups. This, of course, is already clear from what I have said about the difference between affirmation as a method, and affirming living.

Finally, there has to be an increasing amount of sharing of emotions in the process of learning to be a healthy "emotional," sensitive, feeling person. Generally, this sharing of emotions can begin sooner with the nonassertive emotions, than with the emotions of anger, irritation, annoyance, hate and dislike. This sharing, too, must be regulated and directed by the laws of gradualness, human nature, and divine laws. This is particularly important for the feelings which are so easily abused because of their pleasurable aspects: the sexual feelings, and the desires for food and drink.

"The more necessary something is, the more the order of reason must be preserved in it,"[29] is a particularly apt quotation in reference to the sex drive. For the very reason that sexual power is so necessary for the survival of the race, and the desire for food and drink for good health, they need the preserving and defending order of reason. This needs no further explanation in a society which presents such ample evidence of what happens when this fundamental truth is denied and ignored.

In conclusion, a few helpful maxims:
1. Being honest and spontaneous with all your emotions

and feelings, under the ready, natural guidance of a well-informed reason and a well-oriented will, perfects the relationship with yourself, others and God. A well-developed emotional life is indispensable to a satisfying, fruitful spiritual life.

2. If your new, mature ways of responding to your angry feelings cause you to lose a friend, then your friendship with that person was not a true friendship, but a state of neurotic dependency. Sharing your true feelings, also those of anger, in mature ways never kills love and friendship. It deepens and strengthens a basically healthy relationship.

3. The advice of "forgive and forget" is good. The complaint of many people that it "doesn't seem to work for them" is evidence that it requires special clarification in the light of what I have said about the nature of our emotions in general, and the emotion of anger in particular.

Q. Dr. Baars, I am particularly interested in healing through prayer. Would your discussion of the need for forgiveness be a good time to touch on this topic? More and more people are resorting to prayer for their need to be healed.

A. Yes, it would. The spiritual aspects of psychological healing constitute an essential part of any discussion on healing. I am most impressed by what I have observed and learned in my contact with leaders in Christian renewal and prayer movements. It is to be hoped that more professionals in the fields of medicine, surgery and psychiatry become open to how faith and prayer can contribute to their specialties. They may be hesitant to do this because of the fact that the Catholic charismatic renewal and Protestant pentecostal movements seem to have attracted so many people with emotional afflictions. However, this phenomenon, resulting from the therapeutic failures of the young specialty of psychiatry, should not be a deterrent, but rather an invitation to the professions, to investigate with impartiality how the teachings of Christ can complement and perfect its secular concepts and work on behalf of the sick.[30]

As long as I have been engaged in bringing understanding regarding the topic of anger, I want to conclude this first by a discussion of forgiveness. Following this I want to add a few remarks about certain aspects of healing through prayer.

When do we forgive the person whose offensive behavior—his betrayal, his manipulations, his taking advantage of us—has aroused our anger and resentment? The answer to this question is provided by what I have said about the function of anger and all other emotions. Our anger arouses us to respond in the most effective way to the anger-provoking situation. We must first explore and apply every reasonable way to defend ourselves, to be reconciled, to obtain justice, to convince the offending person that he needs to correct his wrongdoing, that he must make restitution. For that God gave us the *psychic motor* of anger, and the "steering mechanism" of reason and will.

When everything reasonable has failed to give us our just due, and we cannot but continue to feel anger and resentment, the time has come to consider the solemn deed of forgiveness. Only then, and not before. For in this matter it is equally true that:

There is an appointed time for everything, and a

time for every affair under the heavens. (Eccles.
3:1)

There is a time to forgive, and a time not to forgive.
The reason I can say this is because some people harm
themselves by "premature forgiveness," which is
detrimental to their psyche, even when moved by the
holiest of intentions. Some people forgive prematurely in
order not to have to face their feeling of anger. Being
accustomed to repression of what is for them an
unacceptable emotion, there is nothing left for
them—when possessed of good will and a desire to obey
God's laws—but to forgive. But these are precisely the
persons who will complain that they cannot forget even
though they have forgiven. They then usually blame
themselves for the persisting feelings of anger and
resentment which in turn keep the memories alive of the
injustices and offenses committed against them.

The "premature forgivers" will often accuse
themselves of not having "really" forgiven the offender, of
not having been sincere, of being bad Christians. They
become confused and bewildered because for them the
maxim "to forgive is to forget" does not apply. Some
extend this idea to God and assume that He, too, does not
forget their sins, even though He has indeed forgiven
them. What is caused by a psychological malfunction,
namely premature forgiving, is interpreted in moral
terms, and leads to self-condemnation, guilt feelings,
weakening of faith in God. The dangers of depression and
despair are ever present, as well as the other
consequences inherent in a neurotic way of living.

By erring to the other extremes, that is by refusal to
forgive, or not forgiving out of ignorance in this matter, a

person will suffer equally untoward consequences. His feelings of anger and resentment, if not bitterness, will grow in intensity and thus increasingly affect his psychic and physical states. It provides the fertile soil in which a psychosomatic disorder can take root, as well as for preoccupation with revenge and self-pity which interfere with one's daily duties, recreation, prayer life, and the joy of living.

The one and only thing that can prevent these adverse developments is the timely act of one's will, namely forgiveness. I am convinced that when Jesus taught us to pray the *Our Father*, He had in mind our psychological well-being as much as our spiritual wholeness. He knew that every one of us would be repeatedly in situations in which he had "every right" to feel anger and resentment as natural reactions to ill treatment by others. Wanting us to be happy even in those circumstances, He gave us—in addition to reason and common sense to be used for the purpose of defense and attainment of justice—the ultimate "tool," so to speak, to be saved from the consequences of chronic, unresolved anger and resentment. That particular "tool," of course, is the act of forgiving.

This wonderful self-help "technique" must be employed in the correct way because it is a special gift of Jesus to us; it must be put to work with His help and participation. As it is an act of the will, and not a matter of feeling, it is done, ideally, only once for one particular offense by one particular person. (Special circumstances may make it necessary, of course, to forgive more than one person, even many, at one time.)

As our emotions, in this case our anger, usually do not immediately "know" what has taken place on the intellectual and spiritual level, they will make themselves felt again after one has forgiven. We still feel resentment even after one has forgiven! This is not proof that we were not sincere when we forgave that person, and asked Jesus to forgive him, too. It is the result of the imperfection of our being in the state of original sin. Our nature lacks the complete unity and wholeness that it possessed originally before the Fall. To the extent and degree that this unity is incomplete—more so in persons with neuroses than in fully affirmed and mature persons—will we experience for a while a resurgence of our anger and resentment after we have forgiven.

When this happens we can accelerate the ultimate quieting of these feelings by asking the Lord to bless that person whom we have and He has forgiven. A short prayer to that effect, while visualizing that person as our brother or sister in Christ and loved by Him, said each time our resentment makes itself felt, will assure the ultimate disappearance of our anger and resentment. The memory of what has happened will no longer disturb us because the Lord has healed us of its pain. Christ, the Healer, has done what no psychiatrist or psychologist can do under those circumstances. No drug, no electroshock treatment, no advice to "forget it; there is nothing you can do about it at this late date," can undo or eliminate traumas of this sort. The Christian therapist knows this and aids his patients who have chronic resentments and psychosomatic afflictions by familiarizing them with the therapeutic instrument of forgiveness.[31]

Q. I appreciate this way of interrelating the psychological and spiritual aspects of our nature. It has obvious practical applications that should appeal

to every therapist. Can you expand a little more about the healing aspects of the charismatic and pentecostal movements in our society?

A. "A little" is all that space will permit here. The subject matter is too vast to do it justice here. Suffice it to say that there are significant things happening among Christians who work at renewing the Church and the lives of the people of God.

What attracted me most to the charismatic renewal was the absence of the fear of the Lord, and the joy the members felt and manifested in sharing their prayer life together in Jesus. Their hunger for the Word of God and their openness to guidance by the Holy Spirit often have a remarkable effect on their personal lives. There is a greater spontaneity and sharing of feelings among most charismatics that, not surprisingly, scare off the uninitiated, especially the older generations who were raised in a reserved atmosphere, leading them to distrust man's sensory emotional experiences.

Because there are so many persons with emotional difficulties among charismatics there exists a tendency for unrealistic expectations for healing of these sufferings. No doubt this is somewhat aggravated by the numerous instantaneous healings of physical illnesses that are reported from all over the world. Reports of healing of inoperable cancers, incurable diseases, severe injuries, congenital defects and mental retardation are not infrequent and testify to the infinite power of God's healing love for us.

Although there are claims of similar healings of emotionally and mentally ill people occurring within a very short span of time, I doubt that this occurs very frequently. In my experience the healing of the emotionally ill person takes place gradually and in stages. In my opinion, this is the more gentle and loving way for God to deal with His afflicted children.

A person who has been the victim of a neurosis since childhood would be at a loss as to how to live in a healthy manner if the Holy Spirit suddenly were to heal his neurosis. His lack of experience would be a formidable obstacle. If he were to be surrounded by emotionally full-grown and integrated friends and relatives it might be possible. But as conditions in society are now, the suddenly mature person would have considerable difficulty in convincing others that his way, not theirs, was the truly healthy, normal way of life.

What I do observe frequently, and what I believe is the experience of all prayerful people engaged in inner healing through prayer, is that the Lord heals in stages. He proceeds with healing from one traumatic memory to the next as they are offered to Him for healing in prayer. Or He heals them according to His own wisdom, without direction from the suffering person or his therapist.

In that way there is time for the sufferer to gradually grow emotionally and to adjust to the social and moral demands and obligations associated with a more healthy personality. His friends and relatives in turn have time to adjust to his new way of being in the world, and to learn from him and his newly gained insights and experiences.

In general I would advise those engaged in the healing of memories to de-emphasize effectivity in prayer. By this I mean that they should be less doing-oriented, less reliant on techniques of prayer, being less directive in constructing images of past traumatic scenes to be entered in this or that way by Jesus. Too many prayerful and spiritually gifted people seem to be interested in becoming therapists and counselors and rely more on psychological techniques, than on the one, primary gift essential in all healing prayer: compassion for the sufferer.

It is the affectivity of the heart, one's compassion, that is the primary quality the Lord responds to and uses in His compassionate healing. Time and time again, the healings Jesus did in His lifetime followed directly upon His being moved to tears, with compassion and with the deepest emotions. He used no methods or techniques of psychodrama or positive imagination. Agnes Sanford said that no healings occur without compassion on the part of the person who prays with another. What I have said earlier about the difference between authentic affirming living and pseudo-affirmation applies with equal force to the difference between compassionate healing and techniques of healing through prayer.

This is not to say that the one who prays should not be familiar with psychological and emotional matters as I have described in this book. On the contrary, a sound knowledge of these matters will enable him to quickly grasp the psychological nature of a person's afflictions and their relationship to his spiritual life. These insights will do two things for him. First, they will deepen his compassion for the other and his suffering, and second, they will facilitate his choosing the correct order and timing of praying for the different memories in need of healing.

Man's affectivity, I have indicated before, is always in danger of being stifled by his effectivity. This holds equally true in the area of healing prayer. This precious, but fragile, possession must be protected at all times against the onslaught of our easily stimulated effectivity, which always threatens to put *man* in the center of the healing "movement," rather than *God* who uses our enlightened compassion for our suffering fellow human beings.

In this connection, I want to remind persons engaged in the ministry of inner healing that they *must never probe* for hurts and painful memories. They must be respectful for the need for privacy and not put a person under pressure to reveal himself against his will. They should always keep in mind that it is not important for a therapist or healer to know everything about a sick or distressed person. What is important and therapeutic is that the latter trusts him enough, and feels really confident enough, to share certain intimate and private areas of his life voluntarily.

A final word concerns the need for a better understanding of man's emotional life among charismatics. They have been affected adversely by the substitution in our language of the word "feel" for "think, believe, know," etc. They too do not always know the difference between feeling and knowing, and are confused as to the origin of their beliefs and attitudes. It seems plausible that their often observed fear of making judgments, and excessive reliance on inspiration by the Holy Spirit in making even the simplest decisions, is related to this confusion.

It seems more logical to assume that the Holy Spirit wants charismatics to *use* all the God-given tools and faculties of their nature, rather than *substitute* the inspiration of the Holy Spirit for them. Besides, what faculties would be left under those conditions to determine what is from the person himself, and what from the Holy Spirit?

I am glad to see a gradual change for the better in the attitudes of charismatics and their understanding of human emotions. There is some better teaching on this topic, though there is still quite a way to go before this will become universal throughout the charismatic renewal. I base my comments on teachings originating in what is generally considered to be the center of the Catholic charismatic renewal in North America, and made available on tape cassettes.[32]

While the basic attitude toward our emotions presented in this series is sound, the subject is "spiritualized" too quickly. The author, a well-known pastoral leader, cautions against misreading of the Scriptures which in the past have created an unnecessary fearful and suspicious attitude toward our emotions. There are still obvious traces of this attitude of old in this presentation. "When we surrender ourselves to the Lord, it sets us free over our desires and emotions" suggests that they are not so desirable after all. So does the statement: "To crucify the flesh and its passions happens when we belong to Jesus." They appear to contradict the opening remarks that emotions are not our enemies (like a tiger in the basement). The tapes contain good teachings on humility and guilt, yet they have relatively little to do with emotions as such. Statements like: "Wrong feelings are temptations," "We must learn how to handle anger," "Fear of the Lord is a good form of fear, a high form of fear," detract from the overall value of the series. Nevertheless, these cassettes constitute a good beginning and can be a valuable help in association with a more complete treatise on human emotions.

The main obstacle I have encountered in the therapy of depressed persons—more in fundamentalists than in

Protestants and Catholics in general—is the firm belief that *anger is a sin*. Not long ago a married woman in her late thirties sought treatment for a severe and disabling depression. It had developed insidiously a year earlier not long after she had become a "born-again Christian." She had been raised without religion. For the six months before her visit she had slept twelve to sixteen hours a day, and in her waking hours she ate constantly so that she had become grossly overweight. On her fourth visit she said, "Dr. Baars, I hope you don't mind my saying this, but I have to have complete confidence in you, if I am to do what you tell me. Everything you have said so far about anger makes sense to me, but for me the final word in everything lies in the Bible. It contains many passages that contradict what you have said about the goodness of anger. I have also read several books by good Christians who state clearly that anger is a sin, and that we must rid ourselves of it. Now I am confused and don't know what to do."

I explained to her my concepts about anger in the light of what is recorded in the Scriptures. Most of this is contained in the pages of this book. When she understood that there was no real contradiction, she dared to begin to follow my advice. Her depression lifted in a relatively short time and she became again the reasonably assertive woman she had always been. Her pseudo-neurotic depression had been preciptated as the result of her resolute decision to lead the Christian life and follow its teachings to the letter. Instead of joy, however, it had brought her grief. Without a spiritually oriented therapy, her depression would have deepened in spite of medication, and the risk of eventual suicide would have become considerable.

Q. From time to time one hears about the need for deliverance and exorcism in people with emotional and mental illness. Does this mean that these illnesses can be caused by evil spirits?

A. There was a time when I, not unlike most professionals in the human sciences, would have scoffed at such a possiblility, if it had occurred to me at all. It is not that I have ever lacked belief in the existence of Satan and other evil spirits; there is simply too much evidence in the Scriptures to deny their existence. But I had always considered all forms of psychological illness to be obviously the result of natural causes so that it did not occur to me to give any thought to the likelihood of supernatural forces being involved in the genesis of psychological illness.

However, having witnessed a fair number of deliverances during the past five or six years, I no longer doubt that evil spirits can play some role in the cause or aggravation of psychological disorders, and can exercise an obstructive force to effective therapy. This is not to say that I agree with those persons who hold that evil spirits are responsible for all or nearly all such disorders. There simply is no evidence to support such a contention. It lacks as much proof as the contention of others who categorically disclaim the involvement of evil spirits in any and all psychological and physical disorders.

Because of the fact that the truth lies always in the middle, every professional must keep in the mind the possibility, if not the probability, of evil spirits exerting influence on the psyche whenever a person comes to him for treatment of an emotional or mental illness. At present the diagnosis of a spirit-caused illness must be made largely by exclusion, by the unresponsiveness to all known forms of therapy, and the historical information suggesting introduction and activity of evil forces in the life of the patient or his ancestors. However, once the deliverance process has begun, the presence of evil forces always manifests itself in unmistakable clinical signs and behavior. It is to be hoped that this subject will become the object of serious research by Christian professionals and ministers. Early differentiation and recognition of supernatural forces involving persons with psychological afflictions will make it possible to institute proper approaches to the healing process, thereby shortening the duration of the illness.

Of more immediate relevance to the topic of this book is the observation that many Catholic charismatics and Protestant pentecostals are inclined to consider certain human emotions as evil, because in the process of deliverance spirits often identify themselves as "anger," "lust," "despair," "hate," and so on. On lecturing to fundamentalists and Full Gospel Business Men's Fellowship meetings, I am often asked how I can consider *fear* a good emotion in view of Jesus' repeated admonitions to not be afraid, to "have no fear." While the answer to this and similar questions—which I like to call in a spirit of friendship, "Bible Bullets"—is obvious, the identification of evil spirits with names of emotions demands some reflection.

Since Satan is the father of lies, and his evil spirits cannot be expected to be any better than he is, it seems to me that they are not particularly interested in making sure that we are told the truth. In fact, it would be to their advantage to make us believe that our God-given emotions are actually evil, instead of good and necessary parts of our nature. Apart from the observation that in deliverance we are not always sure whether it is a spirit who speaks when asked to identify himself, or the person himself who lives in the belief that he is an evil person (e.g., because he entertains feelings of anger), it seems reasonable to assume that the spirit would answer with a single word, rather than with what seems to me would be a more accurate description, like "repressed anger that is beyond control by reason and will."

Some years ago I became the "victim" of such a spirit in one of my patients, a woman religious with severe obsessive-compulsive neurosis and deprivation neurosis. In our therapy sessions this woman developed an uncanny ability to arouse my anger. This, of course, is not too uncommon, but what concerned me was my inability to control it. This had never happened before, or since, but in this case session after session ended with a loud exchange of angry remarks and the patient storming out of the room in tears.

Finally, after weeks of my wondering what was happening, and why I could not handle my anger in a calm, professional manner, the sister expressed her own concern with this development in what was once a consistently pleasant, friendly physician-patient relationship. She told me she liked and respected me greatly and had no reason to be angry with me, but she knew exactly what to do or say that would make me lose my temper. It seemed, she added, that there was something in her that made her do or say those things.

With her permission, I consulted Fr. Francis MacNutt, O.P., who happened to visit me around that time. On his recommendation, we prayed over my patient for deliverance. She was indeed delivered of several spirits that left her quietly and without much objection. None of them identified themselves, nor were they instructed to do so, but if one of them had, I am certain it would have used the word "anger." There was a dramatic change in the patient's behavior and appearance from then on. Never again did her words or facial expression reveal any feeling of anger or hate toward me. The therapy sessions regained their calm.

For the benefit of professionals not familiar with the spiritual aspects of healing, I shall conclude this chapter with an account of a most unusual healing. It merits attention because of its excellent clinical documentation, thorough testing, and several years of follow-up by professionals of a scientific rather than a "believing" bent. It involves a psychological disorder that resists all efforts at treatment through psychotherapy.

At the age of twenty-one a transsexual with a "normal male chromosomal pattern, without psychosis, defective judgement or abnormal affect" was fully prepared for sex-reassignment surgery. With facial hair removed by electrolysis, breast enlargement by means of estrogen, and first name change from John to Judy, he was passing well as a female. He had cross-dressed since the age of four. As a favor to a friend of his, he visited, on his way to the clinic to undergo surgery, a "physician of a fundamentalist Protestant religion foreign to his own, nonpracticing Baptist background." Following a total physical exam he was told that "his real problem was possession by evil spirits."

After some discussion of this, there followed a "two to three hour session involving exhortations and prayers by the physician and laying on of hands on John's head and shoulders." With several faintings during this period "twenty-two evil spirits were exorcised which the physician called by name as they left John's body. During and after this session he felt waves of God's love coming over him but was physically drained." The physician wrote to the reporting professionals that he "showed John that his life was a fake and that Jesus could redeem him and that a standard prescription of Scripture readings caused the spirit of the woman in John to disappear."

Immediately after the session John announced that he was a man, discarded his female clothing, and had his long hair cut into a short, masculine style. After two weeks he entertained some doubts about his conversion and again experienced some feminine feelings. He went to a very well known faith healer in another state, and after waiting two-and-a-half hours in line, the praying and laying on of hands began once again. During the next ten to fifteen minutes, "John fainted, regained consciousness, fainted again, and, as he stood up to leave and join the audience, he realized that his breasts were gone."

John was followed for two-and-a-half years after the exorcism and "tests of gender identity and gender role behavior showed a clear reversal of gender identity." He dated ten girls during the next two years, experienced some sexual arousal toward them, but never masturbated or considered sexual intercourse because of his religious beliefs. For the first several months he had some sexual thoughts of males, but attributed these to the devil. He was subsequently free of these homosexual thoughts for two years, and was looking forward to marriage.

The authors concluded their report by stating, "What cannot be denied, however, is that a patient who was very clearly a transsexual by the most conservative criteria, assumed a long-lasting masculine gender identity in a remarkably short period of time following an apparent exorcism." [33]

Chapter 8

Erroneous Goings On

With the "feeling cult" gaining in popularity we witness a growing movement to better the "mental health" of our population. Led by the psychiatric profession, financed and directed by many government agencies, this movement launched a popular auxiliary front of non-, near- and para-professionals rushing to the aid of their emotionally starved and disabled brothers and sisters.

While at present psychiatry finds itself in a crisis of credibility,[34] the opposite is true of psychologism and pop-psychology, judging by the book stores' shelves being packed to overflowing with self-help books, and the like. They purport to help people by teaching them the art of selfishness, to fight their fears, to look out for number one, to pursue loneliness, to create and actualize themselves, to hang loose while growing up absurd, to say "no" instead of "yes," to learn the answers to all the questions they never dared to ask, to pull their own strings, to clarify their values, to have a sexual shakedown, to be effective parents, and on and on.

For those who do not like to help themselves, but prefer to be helped by others, there is a great variety of gurus, facilitators, trainers, counselors, resource persons, behavior modifiers, instructors, group directors, with or without academic credentials, who will show them how to touch and affirm, to scream and assert, to reveal and communicate, to sensitize and desensitize, to show and tell and share, in an abundance of workshops, encounter weekends, marathons or candle-lit meditation rooms.

Whatever good may be contained in these literary offerings and workshops toward the goal of warding off and preventing emotional repression and deprivation seems to be offset, to a greater or lesser degree, by forced provocation of feelings that do violence to the law of gradualness, by naive techniques and methods, incorrect psychological advice, lack of sensitivity, and new "you musts" replacing old "should nots." One is reminded of the old saying, "In the land of the blind the one-eyed man is king." The psycho-babble of the Cyclops leads the blind to the fantasy island of "mental health" where they are to enjoy what no one has yet defined intelligibly.

It is necessary to critically examine these varied overreactions to countless decades of warped ideas and moralistic attitudes toward our emotions and feelings. Their excesses, outright falsehoods and corrupt practices must be eliminated, in order that whatever is good and correct in these attempts to liberate people from their neuroses will be more effective and beneficial. As our society is already showing evidence of contamination by new types of emotional afflictions as the result of these supposedly well-intentioned, but often bungling "therapies," the matter must be considered urgent.

The preceding chapters provide sufficient data for the reader to draw his own conclusions about the extent and kinds of abuse in the area of "mental health" books and practices. Nevertheless, I would like to facilitate the reader's investigation of the good, the bad and the ugly of present-day psychologisms and prescriptions for instant gratification of feelings and desires. To present a complete survey, either of the pop-psychology literature, or the vast array of "feeling therapies," is out of the question. Nobody could possibly read all the self-help books or personally undergo all the "therapies." I shall limit myself to the areas and subjects about which I have received the largest number of inquiries from concerned individuals. When criticizing teachings or practices which, in my opinion, represent bad psychology I shall do so without judgment of personalities or persons. I assume and respect their good will. If in this quick overview, I appear to be ignorant of important aspects of modern pop-psychology that have positive value, I would like to be so informed. I shall make use of it in future writings.

Q. Somehow I get the feeling—or should I say impression or suspicion—that you are critical of pop-psychology because it is advocated by lay people, rather than medical professionals.

A. I appreciate your honesty in sharing your impression. Be assured that I shall not hesitate to include in this critical analysis the ideas and practices of members of the medical, psychiatric and psychological professions as well. Already the impact on society of some of their sexual beliefs and practices is proving itself detrimental.

As their "novel," if not sensational, ideas get easy press coverage in the communication media and on TV talk shows, while opposing views from other professionals are usually relegated to the back pages, their adverse influence grows more or less unchecked.

An example of this development is Dr. David Reuben's philosophy that "maximum copulation frequence and maximum number of orgasms equal sexual fulfillment" and its likely causal relationship to what I, and the majority of medical men and women, consider an unacceptable and novel practice among some members of our profession. I am referring to a peculiar outgrowth of the now popular delusion that sexual restraint is emotionally crippling and unfulfilling—namely, erotic behavior by some doctors with their patients.

According to a 1973 survey, 92 out of 460 Southern California physicians believed that "erotic activity between patient and physician, although they did not engage in it themselves, could be beneficial to the patient." Apparently their comments were directed at thirty-five or so Southern California physicians— psychiatrists, general practitioners, internists, obstetricians and gynecologists, and surgeons—who had sexual intercourse with their patients—not in after-hours love affairs, but during office visits. In presenting the results of this survey, the authors stated that "changes in society, including the proliferation of therapies outside the profession, such as self-awareness, self-realization, sensual and erotic awareness, have their effect in stimulating patients and physicians." My own acquaintance with a few such professionals, including some psychologists, engaging in such practices with their clients supports the contention of one of these authors, "to think, from a clinical standpoint, that one can do effective therapy in a dual relation is pure nonsense."[35]

Similar unethical goings on are reported to take place among psychologists. According to one survey 70 percent of 500 male psychotherapists knew patients or physicians who have engaged in sexual relationships within the therapeutic setting. Some of them "rationalize" their conduct by citing the work of Masters and Johnson of prescribing sex surrogate partners for therapeutic purposes! Quite a few were "depressed and found less and less meaning in their psychotherapeutic work." The psychologists reporting on the "poorly enforced sex ethics code of the American Psychological Association" commented that "many psychotherapists are working through in their practices their own deprivations and deficient parent-child relationships." "Their motivation to become therapists, whether as Ph.D., MS.W., or M.D.—is based upon a value system, i.e., ego gratification, monetary compensation, and power. Power and control have become very important elements in our society."[36]

These comments are most interesting and will remind the reader of what I have said earlier about self-affirming persons. (See *Born Only Once*.) These reports should alert the reader to the necessity of seeking not only professionally qualified therapists but also mature and affirmed individuals who have no need to affirm themselves at the expense of their clients.

Q. I am somewhat puzzled by your critical stance toward modern, liberating attitudes in sexual medicine and sex education in the schools. I read a book by several Catholic theologians who appear to support much of what you criticize and consider psychologically unhealthy. Should you not support what Catholic theologians are teaching?

A. I can understand that you are puzzled by my contradicting what appears to be a large body of proponents of new approaches in "sexual health." Actually, it is impossible to say what percentage of educators, psychiatrists, psychologists, physicians, scientists and theologians are in favor of the new permissive and "anything goes" attitudes toward sexual feelings and behavior. They receive most of the publicity in contrast to those who are considered old-fashioned, conservative and "uptight." But it is not a matter of how many people are in favor of "liberated sex" and such. Basic principles, not polls, determine what is right and healthy.

Furthermore, your question seems to suggest that you believe I have an obligation to support all teachings of Catholic theologians. If so, you are mistaken. Catholic theologians are in the business of thinking and speculating about God, but cannot teach anything unless it is in conformity with the teachings of the magisterium. If you referred to the book *Human Sexuality*, you should know that what they write, suggest, and recommend in that book is certainly contrary to magisterial teaching. It is important for Christians to realize this, if they are to keep their balance in this world of ever changing, often contradictory, opinions and beliefs.

The pastoral guidelines contained in *Human Sexuality—New Directions in American Catholic Thought*—are another example of how the feeling revolution has been able to sway, if not poison, thoughts and beliefs. In essence, these five authors, one of whom is apparently also a certified psychologist, hold that the morality of all sexual acts must be determined by "the principle of creative growth toward integration, i.e., the ability of sexual acts to foster the values of self-liberation, other-enrichment, honesty, fidelity, life-service, social responsibility, and joyousness."

What these authors have done, presumably in their concern to ease the sufferings of the large number of neurotic and emotionally deprived Christians, is to lower and dilute objective moral standards. They did so in the mistaken belief that the commandments and moral laws dealing with sexuality were and are responsible for this suffering, rather than the psychologically deficient ways and timing of presenting the truths of our faith to young people.

Thus these authors, while frankly admitting that "broad consultation from recognized experts in the social and behavioral sciences provided only inconclusive data on the issues of human sexuality," revealed their ignorance of the fundamental distinction between neurotic repression and mature rational guidance of emotions. Yet it is precisely this crucial distinction which provides the key to the prevention and healing of emotional-spiritual afflictions. That this key is sound both morally and psychologically, the five theologians could have discovered for themselves, if they had studied man as man, with all his God-given faculties, and not merely as a behavioral response to environmental pressures.

As the pastoral guidelines offered in the aforementioned book represent, in my opinion, nothing more than *psycho-theological quicksand*, Christian readers are warned not to follow them. Even if they were not to be morally culpable for adhering to those guidelines, because of the seeming authority of their source, they certainly would not escape serious psychic damage.

Still another example of the effect of the corrupt notion that emotions and feelings are of greater importance than thinking and knowing is the rapid deterioration of moral values and behavior in youth. Responsible for this modern indoctrination, directly or indirectly, in my opinion, are the teachings, programs and philosophies offered by Fletcher's *Situation Ethics*, Sidney Simon's *Values Clarification*, Lawrence Kohlberg's *Cognitive Moral Development*, SIECUS' *Sex Education in Schools*, and to a lesser extent Rev. Vincent Dwyer's *Genesis II* of more recent vintage. The common denominator of these modern teaching programs—listed incompletely here—is the awesome value placed on the *process* as over against the *content* of moral thinking and choosing values. The above process of so-called moral thinking is really moral *feeling*. What makes *you* feel good, fulfilled, satisfied, is the criterion of what is moral for *you*, and therefore must be accepted and respected by me and others.

The moral absolutes and traditional values of Judaeo-Christian religions, unfortunately not always taught in times gone by with optimal respect for "process," are being rejected with a vengeance in these modern teachings. The absolutes, taught by a God who is perceived by many as insensitive to our feelings, as demanding, authoritarian, coldly just, testing and scoring our weaknesses, are being thrown out and ignored. Now *our* feelings determine what is right and wrong, and it is how *we* feel relative to this or that course of action that counts. The tyranny of a feeling self replaces the tyranny of an unfeeling God.

God no longer exists, or if He does, is irrelevant, while man is sovereign, a law unto himself, autonomous.

Man no longer can "impose" his morality on others, as there is no moral law that holds true for all. Instead, man imposes his feelings on others, usually called "rights," against which there is no real objection possible. The old dictum, *de gustibus non est disputandum*—one cannot argue about tastes—also holds true for feelings and emotions; they are beyond dispute, they are personal and unique. One can only reasonably argue about ideas and beliefs.

Likewise, my *moral* rights carry with them the corresponding obligations on the part of others to respect them. But this is not true for my *emotional* "rights" or feelings. They might very well conflict directly with those of others. Which will win out can only be determined by force or power; or endless, fruitless, futile attempts to arrive at consensus; or the prolonged legal skirmishes of a society whose "morality is little more than a legalistic system."[37]

Thus "moral indoctrination" is making way for "process indoctrination," and is being justified and made palatable and attractive to thousands of teachers in both public and private schools, C.C.D. coordinators, high school guidance counselors, "social workers," "mental health" professionals, and the like, in our society. A brief outline of two such popular and widespread indoctrinations may be helpful for the uninitiated in understanding similar programs. They may also clarify to the ordinary, nonprofessional people—usually parents whose "only" gift is common sense and a heartfelt knowledge of truth—why they often feel so frustrated and helpless in these changing times.

These two popular programs of "process indoctrination" reveal how their thrust is to teach children to be suspicious of parental authority and values; to insist on their own preferences in all questions of behavior; to prefer comfort, security, instant gratification and survival above all else; and to reject any absolute standards of right and wrong, especially as presented and upheld by institutional churches and religions.

In Sidney Simon's "values clarification"—widely used in elementary and secondary public and private schools—the children's growth, freedom and ethical maturity are promoted by helping them to know what they want, like and dislike. This is done by means of exercises or "strategies" offering choices as to their emotional preferences. For example, a group of children will be presented with the strategy, "What is the most religious thing to do on Sunday: (a) go to church to hear a good preacher; (b) listen to classical music on the radio; (c) have a big breakfast with the family?"

This and similar strategies offer severely limited and misleading options for conduct. As Simon holds that "no one has the right set of values to pass on to other people's children," they are not advised of the importance of knowledgeable, well-informed, and conscientious judgment of moral issues. What matters to Simon is that they become clear about their desires and ways of self-gratification.

This, of course, has a tremendous appeal to the growing number of youngsters in our society whose needs for authentic love and respect have been frustrated by unaffirmed and denying parents. With their starved emotional life these children are all too ready to devour *any* emotional food, unable as they are to distinguish junk food from health food, and unable to appreciate the higher caloric intellectual and spiritual foods.

The more sophisticated ideas of Lawrence Kohlberg's six states of moral development exert their greatest influence on departments of psychology and philosophy and schools of education. Based on the work of Piaget, and certain cultural and anthropological studies, and developed at Harvard and the Center for Moral Education, Kohlberg's concepts can be summarized as follows:

1. Traditional moral education is undemocratic and unconstitutional.
2. What is needed is a new psychology and philosophy that recognizes the child's right to freedom from indoctrination. The child must be seen by adults not as a pupil, but as a "moral philosopher in his own right."
3. By means of exercises involving moral dilemmas and conflicts the child must develop through his "Six stages of cognitive moral development."

With the aid of a text containing twenty-one sexual conflicts and twenty-nine nonsexual ones,[38] students are encouraged to argue and then vote in a democratic fashion, while the teacher remains "impartial, relaxes and enjoys it."

While Kohlberg's theory is supposed to provide an

improved version of Simon's method—the apex of morality, achieved in the sixth stage, is to treat every man impartially according to what is "justice" or "equality"—practice does not square with theory in Kohlberg's universe. As moral judgment to a very large extent involves assessing competing claims of individuals about their rights, their emotional wants, desires and preferences come to override reason, justice and impartiality in the discussion of "moral dilemmas."

We don't have to be educators or pupils to know what Simon and Kohlberg represent. All of us experience in some way or other its tragic consequences: a world made increasingly less attractive by the tyranny of opposing passions and rights of minorities and majorities; by the pressures of the wants of special groups with influence and connections; by a more selfish, immoral, cold and ugly world that knows less and less the freedom of authentic morality, the genuine love, friendship and fidelity for one another founded in a loving God.

Genesis II, a very expensive, time-consuming program of films, tapes, minutely arranged and outlined fun exercises, sensitivity sessions, group discussions, "take-home" paperwork, etc., aims at "trying as a group of friends to discover and experience more realistic meanings of spirituality in our lives." The facilitator's handbook states emphatically that "the intellectual is not stressed in this program," that it is "devoid of formal study," because "sharing insights and experiences and feelings about what it means to be human and Christian" are the principles of spiritual growth.

Steeped in Piaget's and Kohlberg's stages of moral growth, the Trappist originator of this program—"internationally acclaimed for his expertise in the behavioral sciences and their relationship to spirituality"—claims that "feelings are the *best* indicator of what people value, so you must be in touch with your feelings." That the program is also badly in need of a more wholesome understanding of man's emotional life is evidenced by such statements as "expressing your *negative* feelings can also be helpful"; and "positive affirmation" (as if there could be such a thing as negative affirmation).

As in most other "growth-programs," Genesis II sees the process of affirmation as a matter of *doing*, "building a person up," by "giving strokes," avoiding "putting down" remarks; and by a series of "affirmative exercises." A typical example of these mostly childish and boring exercises—for adults, and junior/senior high school students—is that of participants walking around in a room with a sandwich board over their shoulders. On the front of these boards each person has written down what he thinks and feels about himself, while the others are to write down on the back of the board what they feel about him.

For whom this program has been designed is not clear from the Genesis II facilitator's handbook. One gets the impression that it is for emotionally underdeveloped or disturbed Christians, who are thought to be in need of behavioristic programing and possibly also ideological brainwashing. It seems unlikely that any educated Catholic, even if in need of emotional growth, would be willing to complete all eighteen sessions after having been exposed in the fourth to an offensive, shallow, humanistic taped presentation of two views of how God created the world.

Interestingly, it is precisely at this point in the program, after the participants have been made to listen to what some people might well consider a blasphemous "fanciful little skit," that the facilitator is warned to resist any suggestions by the participants that the format be changed, and that they do something else, because "they may be uneasy with the process or may not fully adjust to where it is going and may suggest that someone tell them more"! The group *must* be kept in line with "a light touch, but nonetheless firmly."[39]

I would like to conclude my critique on a positive note. The teachings and practices of Simon, Kohlberg and Dwyer could be put to better use, if their strategies, exercises and games were to *complement* rather than *replace* sound moral teaching. That way the students would learn to distinguish between absolute moral values, subjective moral opinions and their own feeling responses to the persons faced with moral dilemmas. Of course, such a case study approach is far from novel. However, with our present deeper understanding of man's emotional life and its influence on his intellectual life and spiritual life, it would provide an even greater challenge to the casuist of great intellectual acumen and honesty.[40]

The word "affirmation" has become popular this past decade among human relationship and mental health counselors. Every one is speaking of affirmation and trying "to do it" to others. They say there has been precious little of it in the past, and that we must affirm each other if we are to become emotionally mature and happy.

In spite of this good news, proclaimed by so many, there is little evidence of *authentic* affirmation being around. Good will and a sincere desire to improve the shortcomings of past interpersonal relationships, yes, but real strengthening of each other, no.

Interestingly, wherever members of a community—religious, prayer group, covenant—use the term most freely and glibly, there seems to be the least amount of true affirmation. Such places depress one with their bustling activity—planned togetherness, meetings, expected modes of behavior and participation, carefully scheduled recreation, etc. There seems little opportunity for just *being*—even less for being different or for wanting to be alone. Underneath the new freedom of behavior is often a hidden agenda of *new conformism*.

For certain, those who cannot help being different are not expelled. They are tolerated in a kindly, long-suffering way—full of hope and expectation that some day they, too, will want to conform to the *new* way of living. *New* because it differs as night from day from the old way. Not *new* as the result of having grown out of the new heart that God promised He would give His people. The sign of "new heart living" is *communion*; yet, there is still too much *communication* to permit communion and authentic being.

Techniques and methods of pseudo-affirmation flourish everywhere. There is surprisingly little creativeness in these methods, as I see them taught and practiced around the country. At least much less than one would expect to be possible in devising ways of doing, saying, acting, playing with one another. This might well be proof of man's discursive mind having a more limited capacity than his intuitive mind, the true source—together with his humane emotions—of authentic affirmation, of being present to everything created with one's whole being.

Few seem to have delved deeply enough into the meaning of what I decided to call "affirmation" when I first—in the early sixties—translated Dr. Terruwe's term *bevestiging*.[41] It seems an easy concept, so readily understood on first acquaintance. And even if one is told correctly that affirmation is a matter of *being*, not of *doing*, one wants to be practical and begin immediately with doing affirming things for others. Who has the time and patience to wait for the strengthening effect to slowly and gradually grow from another person's way of being-in-the-world? The need for affirmation is too great! One must act at once!

There is another subtle difference between affirmation and pseudo-affirmation. Affirmation, or rather, as I described earlier, affirming living, is a way of being, in fact, the only way of living authentically as a human being, as another Christ. It is fruitful for everyone involved in terms of the highest human values: life, love, psychic health, and happiness.

Affirmation, on the other hand, as a way of doing, is fruitful only, or can be so in the hands of certain people, in terms of utility and gain. It can serve the self-affirmer in eminent ways when employed skillfully in a business-like way. Of course, this can only be done under the banner of "affirmation," for no one wants to buy an *ersatz*—or substitute—product, when the real thing is needed. Though the difference between the real thing and the substitute is clear to the mature, the true thinker, the sensitive one, it is much less so to the ones most in need of the real stuff. And because it is better than the stuff of denial that has caused the deepest wounds in the unaffirmed, the crumbs of pseudo-affirmation can be mistaken for real health food. But only for so long. In time, one will realize that health and happiness and healing are not forthcoming. Just as the prisoner in a concentration camp, or Gulag, will devour ravenously the watery "soup" to prolong his life, only to realize in time that it is ebbing away, and that all he has gained is time, and maybe hope, for eventual liberation.

There are people who have been treated for years—at great expense—in institutes or homes that have the word "affirmation" in their logo, who are unable to tell me in what way those places were different from those not claiming to offer affirmation therapy.

They were given individual and group counseling, medications, psychodrama sessions and the like while living together in home-like settings, yet they had never felt a special, healing force emanating from the staff members, who directed them, but who were never a real part of their lives. Though things looked different, and were given special names, it was the usual story of staff versus clients, of professionals who do not live the affirming life, but at certain times, in certain situations, push the button of affirmation (i.e., pseudo-affirmation), and expect great things to happen. But they do not. They only happen when a person lives for a while in the orbit of others who live the affirming life!

This is not to say that there are no such life-giving, others-strengthening communities. There are places—not necessarily professional or therapeutic institutes—where people really share and bear each other's burdens and joys in prayerful, truly unselfish ways, unconcerned about material gains and acquisition of reputation or fame. But, as far as I know, none of them employ the word "affirmation" in their logos.

All this goes to show that those who live the authentic affirming life have no need to talk about it. Their way of living does the talking! Jesus led this life. His apostles learned it by osmosis; they were fulfilled by living in the orbit of the First Authentic Affirmer.

Again, a positive note is in order. Techniques and methods of so-called affirmation have their value in helping people to relinquish their various ways of denial of other persons. Denial, the very opposite of affirmation, has been around a long time, and has left a long trail of psychic wounds in its wake. However, we should not dignify these methods of teaching more constructive ways of relating with the label of affirmation. To designate methods of increasing sensitivity, human awareness and relations, and personal growth as affirmation represents a form of spoiling. It leads people to believe that there is nothing more to human relationships than being nice and saying and doing the right things. It stifles their desire for learning the authentic way of living, and thus deprives them of the joy of ever experiencing its fruits.

Assertiveness training is one area in which unfamiliarity with the function of our psychic motors, and also with the syndrome of the unaffirmed person, can have adverse consequences for the trainee.

Assertiveness-training programs are a sophisticated outgrowth of the psychiatrist's advice to his passive, unassuming patient with depression to "go out and get good and mad at some people, break some bottles, or hit golf balls." Probably because of the rapidly rising number of meek and subdued persons, and with the growing interest in feelings and emotions, certain people saw their way clear to advance themselves by training people to develop their "aggressive drive." Mostly in groups, people's emotions of anger were force-fed by a variety of stimuli, for the purpose of letting them erupt. They were congratulated and encouraged, of course for a fee, to continue with these sessions, in the expectation that practice would make perfect, and thereby change the person irreversibly from being meek to having fortitude.

The rapid rise and fall of the assertiveness training fad already suggests by itself that all is not well with this approach. Psychologically, there are two basic reasons why this approach does not have beneficial results.

Emotions cannot be forced. As most people are afraid of their angry feelings and of the effect on others if they are to express these feelings, they can only bring themselves to respond to the tactics of the trainer and the group members, by repressing their fear of their anger (just as the meek patient could only obey his psychiatrist's advice by repressing his fear of his anger). But this means that he is trained to behave in a certain—for others—desirable way by means of a neurotic mechanism. In fact, his cooperation is brought about by a *double neurotic repression* (i.e., his prior "single" neurotic repression of anger by fear is "doubled" by the person using his energy to repress the fear that repressed the anger). Instead of improving psychically the person gets worse, even though his assertive behavior pleases the trainer and the group.

If, following the course, the person reverts back to his original passivity and mildness, it is most likely blamed on his not really wanting to be healthy, not having fully cooperated, or of enjoying secondary gains of his unassertive attitude. The real reason, of course, that this training can never "take," is that all neurotic processes in time become inadequate in holding repressed material locked in the subconscious. The energetic repression of the fear of anger, superficial as it is in most assertiveness-training programs, soon proves to be inadequate, and the temporarily repressed fear of anger rises to the surface and makes the person unassertive again.

If, however, the program does take and the previously unassertive person is successfully trained to be assertive, the results are not necessarily beneficial for society. This is particularly true for the unaffirmed trainee. The unaffirmed person whose realistic fear of the adult world keeps him from being himself is not really afraid of his angry feelings (or any of his other emotions). He just wants to be loved by all and therefore learns to be nice and please people (which in their minds excludes "getting" angry). This unaffirmed person, therefore, with good assertiveness training methods can be made to become assertive and abandon his previously too passive and submissive role. If this change in behavior occurs without simultaneous adequate and authentic affirmation of this unaffirmed person, the unaffirmed or deprivation neurotic person is helped to shift to the other side of the spectrum of nonaffirmation, namely to the self-affirming side. While first a meek, self-effacing unaffirmed person, he now becomes an assertive, if not aggressive, self-affirming, unaffirmed person. As I have already discussed the personality of the self-affirming person and his adverse effects on society, the reader realizes that his responsiveness to assertiveness training will not make the world a better place in which to live—neither for others, nor for himself.

In conclusion, assertiveness training programs should not be conducted save by fully mature and affirmed people who know which clients are passive and "meek" because of repression, and which because of lack of affirmation. In addition to this knowledge they should be able to guide the former slowly and gradually to abandon his fear (see chapter 7), and to affirm the latter, whose assertiveness will then spontaneously emerge in his own "untrained" way, and at his own pace.

From time to time I am asked what I think of such self-help organizations as Alcoholics Anonymous, Recovery, Inc., Marriage Encounter, and T-Groups (the model for human awareness, personal growth and sensitivity groups). My commentary on these organizations should probably not be included in this chapter on erroneous goings on, because I consider their positive contributions—except for T-Groups—to outweigh the negative ones.

Alcoholics Anonymous, in stressing a spiritual awakening—"that only a Power greater than the alcoholic can restore him to sanity"—has become the most successful organization to arrest the disease of alcoholism. In living the twelve steps and helping others to live them too, alcoholics assist one another in staying dry. That A.A.'s recovery rate is not higher than it is, stems, in my opinion, from insufficient psychological help from professional sources. A.A.'s *will-training* is excellent in the initial stage which requires the alcoholic to give up alcohol, so he can participate intelligently in the program. However, its educational program relies too much on building up will power, and not enough growth and healing of the emotional life, to assure permanent sobriety. I believe that A.A.'s present recovery rate could be increased by at least 50 percent, if A.A. were to incorporate professional treatment of the alcoholic's underlying psychological difficulties. Why this is not done I have attempted to explain in my article, "The Alcoholic Priest," excerpts of which are contained in the footnote section.[42]

The foregoing comments concerning excessive reliance on will power are also pertinent to Recovery, Inc. Over the years I have treated several leaders of this organization who, in their own words, "had benefitted immensely from the Recovery program," yet had reached a plateau of partial well-being they were unable to transcend.

The core of the program is systematic training of the will, while intellectualizing is taboo. Neither religion nor major moral questions—notably those pertaining to sex—are discussed. All discussions, presented in a format developed by Dr. Low to prevent "debate" and "argument," are limited to the "trivialities of inner environment." Recovery's overall aim is to help clients of psychiatrists to cope in their normal milieu (i.e., to perform in an average manner).

To comment on Recovery's understanding and attitude toward emotions and feelings would lead me too far afield. Suffice it to say that the Recovery clients who sought my help were "startled" by my particular approach. All experienced considerable difficulty in letting up on their attempts to attain *Mental Health Through Will-training*,[43] as they had done for ten to twenty years in Recovery. As a result, their therapy progressed much more slowly and none attained the necessary freedom to be themselves and enjoy the potential contributions of their emotional lives to the fullest.

In my opinion, it would be very difficult, if not

impossible, to integrate the principles of Dr. Low's therapy and those of mine, because the practical effect of the Recovery concept is to promote, rather than eliminate, the process of neurotic repression through will-training.

Marriage Encounter recognizes that its program is not for persons with emotional difficulties. For couples who already have a reasonably healthy and good marriage it offers something of positive value.

However, there is one warning I should sound. In the focus on feelings it is not explained how participants' emotions are to be integrated with their higher faculties, and used in their determination to adhere to the teachings of the magisterium. As it is stated in Marriage Encounter's manual for the couples and priests who present the encounter weekends, "Feelings are personal, inner reactions and are neither right nor wrong. . . . We don't want this talk to be instructional, heavy or lengthy. . . . We aren't teaching about feelings as much as we're sharing the importance we've found sharing them has had in our marriage."[44]

Undoubtedly, this educational void is responsible for the most frequently heard comment to the effect that the couples' emotional growth is not matched by an equal growth in knowledge of employing emotions in the service of adhering to established moral standards. This comment seems to be made most often in reference to the encyclical *Humanae Vitae*.

Correction of this fault of omission would, in my opinion, make this movement one of the most promising contributions by the Church in its effort to build a stronger and healthier family life and to rear emotionally and morally better-equipped children.

The reputation of T-Groups has suffered because of certain excesses. These excesses apparently stem from Western man's mentality to want to speed up and exaggerate a good thing, in order to get even better and bigger results.

If sharing of feelings in groups is of therapeutic value for the participants, then constant hugging, kissing, touching, feeling and the like must have greater therapeutic value. If adults are to express all their feelings, even their sexual ones, then fornication must provide the ultimate means of therapeutic growth. And if this is good for adults in groups, then it must be good also in all life situations and at nearly every age level. If openness and self-disclosure in groups is good, then total and instant self-revelation by discarding all clothing must be better. If involvement of the group participants for a few hours has value, then marathon sessions must have twice as much value.

These excesses are most deplorable from a moral viewpoint, and are psychologically damaging to all participants, not just those with emotional disorders. Unless these excesses are eliminated, unless T-Group leaders are chosen for their professional qualifications, personal maturity and moral character, unless T-Group use is restricted to purposes of training group therapists and of providing an additional treatment modality for wisely chosen patients, and professional psychiatric follow-up of individual participants is provided, I could not recommend such therapy groups.

A presentation of erroneous goings on would be incomplete without mention of the new "sexual freedom." The changes wrought by the revolt against old sexual mores, familiar as they are to all of us, are almost beyond belief.

In less than half a century sexual hang-ups have been replaced by a "liberated" ideology of sex; sexual neuroses by impotence and orgasmic dysfunctions even in young adults; castration anxiety by performance anxiety; shame by sexual prowess; modesty by group sex; premarital abstinence by peer pressure to be sexually active; the tyranny of past "you must not" in matters of sex by the tyranny of "you must"; neurotic repression of sexual feelings by neurotic repression of fear of sex; the old myth that masturbation causes mental retardation by the new myth that it is more fulfilling than intercourse; the birds and the bees by explicit sex "education" and pornography; and post-coital rapture by post-coital depression.

The immediate consequences of the sexual revolution—skyrocketing cases of venereal disease, unwanted pregnancies, crimes against the unborn child, sexual promiscuity, sex crimes, etc.—are overshadowed by the growing deterioration of interpersonal relationships and their widespread effects on society. Casual sex, fun sex and impersonal sex—*all forms of self-affirmation*—have brought alienation and hostility between the sexes; aggravation of feelings of rejection, inadequacy, failure, loneliness and depression; doubled the number of divorces and family breakdowns, of abandoned and battered children; and an alarming rise in suicide rates in young people, especially in the age groups of ten to fourteen and twenty to twenty-four.

That the sexual revolution has been able to spread like

wildfire is due in large part to the constantly growing number of unaffirmed people in our society. Their frustrated need for authentic love makes them extremely vulnerable and makes them put their faith in the false promises and unrealistic claims of sex "educators" who have divorced sex from its procreative purposes and thus from its protective guidance of unselfish love. The psychic trauma inflicted repeatedly by successive discoveries that free sex is not accompanied by affirming love is devastating and further weakens already undeveloped psyches. They either become sexual self-affirmers who inflict their cancerous destruction on others, or commit suicide in despair of never finding what is obviously possessed by persons who are truly in love and dedicated to each other.

While it is true that the old repressive sexual morality derived from distorted notions of human sexuality, the modern notions are even worse. Unfortunately, these modern, perverted concepts of human nature and human sexuality are likely to be with us for some time to come, unless the common sense of ordinary people prevails over the scientific indoctrinations by members of the professions. Influential *sexologists in the medical profession* convened in Geneva in 1974 under the auspices of the World Health Organization Family Health Section. These men and women physicians:

1. Defined sexual health as "the integration of somatic, emotional, intellectual and social aspects of sexual being in ways that are positively enriching and that enhance personality, communication and love";
2. Held that "every person has the right to

receive sexual information and to consider
accepting sexual relationships for pleasure as
well as procreation," and prided themselves on
this "concept of health that is almost
revolutionary!";
3. Were "developing techniques to integrate
human sexuality into health practice";
4. Claimed that "being human means that we
have the privilege of choosing when, how, and
with whom we shall be sexual. This sexual
self-determination is clearly what sex education
is all about."[45]

This "revolutionary sexual health" philosophy is but the
logical outcome of minds that refuse to recognize man as a
spiritual being and deny the validity of objective moral
norms. Moreover, it betrays their ignorance of a
philosophy of human sexuality that presents a
satisfactory alternative to past and present
obsessive-compulsive preoccupation with genital
sex—the past in repressing sex at all cost, the present in
gratifying it by all means. Neither form of sexual
preoccupation has been able to secure the joy and
happiness that is sought by all. One made man neurotic,
the other blunts the feeling of love together with the other
humane emotions, and thus makes him less humane and
his sexual activities less authentically human.

Because the *center of human sexuality* is not located in
our genital organs, but in the brain, it follows that our
intellectual grasp of sexual matters must be correct and
complete. This can be accomplished only if all dimensions
of man's nature are included. No matter how much certain
sexologists and theologians agitate against "moral

imperatives" they hold responsible for sexual neuroses, a philosophy of human sexuality *must* take into account the whole of man, precisely his spiritual dimension. When this is done and the psychological dimension is clearly understood, it is possible to arrive at a philosophy of human sexuality, and of man and woman, that can liberate us from the tyranny of sexual fear and compulsive sexual gratification.

One of the simplest and most lucid presentations of this philosophy can be found in a small sixty-five-page book entitled, *How Can a Man and Woman be Friends?*[46] It is a practical guide to authentic sexual freedom and the joy of authentic love for anyone desirous of finding these in friendship, marriage, or the freely chosen celibate life. It is also must reading for those who want to free themselves from the loneliness and joylessness that is intrinsic to open marriages, casual sex, sexual exploitation, in short, *sex without self-restraining love*.[47]

In conclusion, I want to briefly comment on the common denominator of the aforementioned and other contemporary erroneous goings on. In essence, this consists of a lack of balance between emotional and intellectual affirmation, between the giving of emotional health food and intellectual truths. If one gives too much of one and too little of the other, one always detracts from the value of what is given in abundance. If one gives the emotional health food together with insufficient intellectual and spiritual food, the emotions are denied the necessary internal guidance and tempering. If, on the other hand, one gives an abundance of intellectual and spiritual truths together with emotional junk food, one offers only half-truths. As St. Augustine said, "*Res tantum cognoscitur, quantum diligitur*," "A thing is known to the extent that it is loved." If one's emotional life is undeveloped or repressed, so will be one's capacity to love what is taught.

When Freud's brilliant discovery (that repression of feelings and emotions always causes a neurosis) became public knowledge earlier in this century, concerned educators rushed in to remedy the situation. The insight that the feelings of young people should not be repressed was translated into the maxim that "feelings should not be hurt" or interfered with, and that children should be allowed to "go through a phase." In the home this led to *permissiveness* on the part of the parents, in the school to the *lowering of educational standards* and requirements to the level of the slower and intellectually less gifted students. As great care was taken not to hurt the feelings of the slower students, the brighter ones were not challenged intellectually. They became bored and began to seek other outlets for their feelings and frustrated energies. Both school and home sacrificed their children's innate need for discipline and order by giving them an unbalanced diet of emotional-intellectual-spiritual health food, for fear they would be repressing or hurting their feelings.

Feelings and emotions were increasingly viewed as people's most precious possession, witness the slogan of the unaffirmed person, "I do not want to hurt anybody's feelings!" This precious possession therefore had to be protected just as much as various laws protected their lives against potential murderers, their material possessions against burglars, and their reputation and good name against slanderers. Lacking such direct legal protection against trauma to feelings, permissiveness and sliding standards were here to stay with us for a long time.

We are all acquainted with the disastrous effects on individuals and society of the well-intentioned but too hastily conceived efforts by educators to contribute to the "mental health" of young people. The cure has proved worse than the disease. The juvenile courts are unable to handle the thousands of delinquents arrested each year; the schools have a hard time to teach the three R's and consequently, they graduate relative illiterates; the young seek to dull the pain of emotional and intellectual deprivation in drugs and sexual promiscuity; many abandon sooner or later the religions of their parents, some of them in favor of religious groups or sects where they can find more acceptance and love. To them religious doctrine is less important than the humane qualities of the leaders and the feeling of belonging that membership brings.

Seeking religious affiliation under these circumstances is for most persons, because of their extreme psychic vulnerability, a two-edged sword. Unaffirmed people can be readily taken advantage of by unscrupulous persons in positions of authority. They can be made to live by strict, even harsh, rules and to make financial sacrifices, as long as this guarantees them a certain sense of belonging. In the most extreme cases this may lead to the Jonestown massacre or other destructive consequences.

Protection against such tragic developments and correction of existing inadequacies and shortcomings in education and child rearing can be realized in the future only if we understand and live the basic principles of what I have described in this book as affirming living—the properly balanced emotional, intellectual, spiritual strengthening of our brothers and sisters in the Lord.

Chapter 9

Binds and Disputations

Q. Dr. Baars, I am not sure whether I can square all of your teachings about man's sense of emotional life, interesting as they are, with Scripture. At least not with those passages which I have always interpreted as being condemnatory of man's lower nature. For example, in Romans 8:7, we are told: "The outlook of the lower nature is enmity with God; it is not subject to the law of God; indeed it cannot be: those who live on such a level cannot possibly please God" (NEB). And Romans 8:3 reads: "Because our lower nature robbed it [the law] of all potency" (NEB). Are these passages not a clear indication that our lower nature is a serious source of sin?

A. They seem to be at first glance, I admit. But on deeper reflection it is not hard to see that all of Romans, dealing with this topic, confirms what I have presented in this book concerning the "flesh" and the "spirit." Paul makes it clear that the feelings we possess on the level of our lower nature are not subject to sin and guilt in themselves, only when they are deliberately taken up as an existential position. Only when they and they alone determine our mode of living are the emotions a vehicle of sin. But, even then, it is not they but the freely willed refusal of the will informed by reason to guide the emotions which is the actual source of sin.

Paul's statement that "our lower nature robbed it [the law] of all potency" seems to confirm what I have said about irrational fear and excessive energy interfering with the necessary and needed cooperation between flesh and spirit. These supercharged, utilitarian emotions in the obsessive-compulsive neurotic take over the function of the free will, and thus rob the law given to us by God as a help, not a hindrance, of its willed effect. They make those neurotics impotent before the demands of the law.

The same applies to Romans 7:5: "While we lived on the level of our lower nature [before we were given faith], the sinful passions evoked by the law worked in our bodies" (NEB). Again this is clarified by my thesis on the cause of repressive neuroses. The law, holy in itself, but presented prematurely, or without proper explanations, to young children, stimulates fear or energy which causes repression. The repressed emotions as a result, are denied rational guidance and in time start to operate by themselves in an obsessive-compulsive (i.e., *nonfree*) manner. The "sinful passions"—excessive irrational fear or energy—"evoked [stimulated] by the law," led to objectively sinful behavior.

Q. You say that our emotions are not sins. How can I

feel hate and resentment and unlawful desire and not be sinning?

A. If God punished us for our emotions—instruments of our God-given nature just like our eyes, tongue, fingers—He would be a very unfair God indeed. To restate what I have discussed before: There are two major errors about emotions. One sees them all as sins, to be fought against, because they are of our lower nature. The other sees emotions as the basis of *all* value and *all* action, without reference to any objective good or moral law. This second error is very popular in our time, and, as I discussed in Chapter 8, has produced already most unhealthy consequences.

Rational Christian psychology teaches that our emotions are morally neutral; how we choose to act upon them determines our culpability.

Jesus, fully God, and fully man, and without sin, experienced emotions and feelings which many people think of as sinful. He felt hate toward evil and toward the lukewarm and the moneychangers and the Pharisees. He felt irritation with His disciples, at their lack of faith, their incomprehension, their fears. Moreover, Jesus couches much of His teaching in terms of desires of the human heart and the human body. He never condemns desire, but condemns lust, a willed action with the intention to do wrong (the same applies for the other six "capital sins"—all movements of the will, not emotions). Nor does He ever represent love and forgiveness as mere emotions, but always as *actions* to be willed and performed.

Remember, Jesus loves us and knows us as men and women; He wants us to be renewed and transformed by His grace but as men and women, as human beings, not as perfectly programed robots devoid of free will. He affirms the basic goodness in sinners and shows His faith in them—in Mary Magdalene, the good thief, and many others. The pattern is always the same: first recognizing and revealing to the person his goodness; then the forgiveness and healing of the body and spirit; then and only then, the admonition to go and sin no more. Sin is a deliberate choice, not a feeling; if sin were a feeling, many of the psalms, which express anger and hate, would be sinful.

Q. I always thought we were supposed to get away from the body, and become more spiritual. If I start paying more attention to my emotions and bodily feelings, won't I become less spiritual?

A. This is a common error because there is so much covert Gnosticism in our culture (as there always is in times of intellectual exhaustion or decadence!). The Gnostics taught that the human body is the source of evil in man, and that he must free the spirit from its evil influence. *Body hatred* has its polar opposite in *body worship*, one of the extreme errors of our time. These two opposites tend to generate each other (i.e., Puritanism breeds liberationism, and vice versa).

The psychological manifestations of this constant struggle are very evident in our daily lives. As Christians, we believe in the resurrection of the body, in the Incarnation, and in the goodness of the works of God's creation. At the same time, we believe in the Spirit, the body as the temple for the Spirit, and in the spiritual nature of material creation.

The Gnostics, some of them, taught that Christ could not have a real body, since the body was evil. Jesus refuted them in His resurrected body by cooking and eating fish for breakfast with his friends as the perfect sign of His incarnate reality.

This back-and-forth struggle between body and spirit is futile. It is not body *or* spirit, but body *and* spirit, interacting by means of intellect and emotions (psyche), which enable us to love God. Although the terminology is somewhat different from Paul, this tripartite composition of man is taken directly from the epistle to the Romans, Chapters 7-9, and elsewhere in all his epistles, which serve as the very basis for authentic Christian anthropology. Unless the body, "mind," "heart," and spirit work together, man cannot "Love the Lord [his] God with all [his] heart, with all [his] soul, with all [his] mind, and with all [his] strength" (Mark 12:30 NEB).

Remember also this, Jesus said, "This is my body to be given for you" (Luke 22:19). If Jesus means what He says, and I believe He does, then we can see deeper meaning in this statement from the psychological point of view. I cannot give something to someone unless I fully possess it; I cannot give something with any meaning unless I know it, love it and own it. So Jesus cannot commit the perfect act of love by giving us His body in Communion or crucifixion unless He fully accepts it as His body and loves it for the masterpiece of God which it is.

I cannot fully love in married love unless I can give myself wholly to the other person, which requires that I be in full possession of myself, in the sense that I am not afraid of my body or my emotions and bodily feelings.

The same is true in friendship and the freely chosen celibate life. Here, too, one must be able to give and love freely in self-restraining love (i.e., one must love the friend and all others on all levels of one's being, while restraining oneself in those manifestations of love which do not constitute a good for the other or are contrary to the moral laws). This highest form of human love also requires that one is in full possession of oneself, for what one does not truly possess one cannot readily and joyfully hold back; one cannot have control of something—or freely hold back or let go—unless one possesses it.

A parallel truth is evident in asceticism, the practice of self-denial for the purpose of growing in spirit (such as fasting). This tends to become neurotic when the person is not at home with his body. The point of asceticism is not to hate the body or wish it out of existence, but to point the body in the right direction, in the sense that Paul speaks of it in Romans. As Augustine rightly pointed out, sin, in the teaching of Paul, is evil because of its direction away from loving God. There is a right direction of body, feelings and emotions toward God, all of which can be accomplished only by the person who is fully free to choose that right direction.

Q. I was raised a Catholic and the nuns taught us that we must suffer and offer our sufferings to God. You seem to be saying that we should not suffer, but feel joy and happiness. To me, it sounds as if you are recommending a deviation from the imitation of Christ, and your teaching sounds like all those other psychiatrists who tell us to be free and do as we like.

A. The answer to this apparent contradiction lies in the words of Christ who never taught a beatitude of illness, and in His life that apparently was free of physical, emotional and mental illness. But He did tell us to take up our cross as He did himself, the cross of being misunderstood, hated, persecuted, tortured and put to death. To be able to do so gladly in imitation of Jesus, we need strength, courage, faith, and if at all possible, good health, especially psychic health. For having to share in carrying Jesus' cross while one is physically and/or psychically ill, is more than many people can bear, more than Jesus himself had to bear.

The Christian who becomes ill rightly seeks to be cured by a physician. He will employ every reasonable means to attain physical, emotional and mental health. He makes this suffering redemptive while seeking a cure, and being healed. The same holds true for the suffering of illness for which no cure is possible.

So the nuns were right when they told you: "We must suffer and offer our sufferings to God," but not in the sense you understood it (and, possibly, they themselves meant it). All men must suffer to the extent that suffering of some kind is unavoidable in this unperfect world. But this is not to say that God created us for the purpose of making us suffer. What God had in mind when He created us is obvious from the facts as recorded in Genesis. He created Adam and Eve perfect as human beings, who walked and talked with Him in perfect surroundings called paradise. That their original perfect happiness came to an end as the result of their sin could not have changed God's purpose in creating man. God's purpose continues to be the same: to give all men and women the opportunity to share in His own infinite happiness if they so freely will it.

This is confirmed in the answer to the first question in the *Baltimore Catechism,* "Why are we in this world?" "We are in this world to *know* God, to *love* Him, to *serve* Him, and to be happy with Him forever in the world hereafter."

I admit that this answer implies, at least to some, that

we are in this world for His sake, not for our own, and that we must work hard to please Him by studying, loving and serving Him; and also that happiness is not to be ours now, but only in the world hereafter.

But if we interpret this answer in the light of what I have said about affirming living, and, of course, of all of revelation, we realize that God wants us to be happy and joyful here on earth. For we can come to *know* God only by *being* ever more *present to Him* with the full attention of our whole being; when we do so we will *be moved* with the joy of His love and *love* Him in return; and when we *reveal* to others how moved with joy we are, how much love we feel for Him in himself, and in Him as He is in others, we serve Him. But again, in our serving others this way, we often will be loved in return, and we experience with them also the joy of love. The lasting joy of the life hereafter then becomes the ultimate fulfillment of our capacity for joy and happiness as we have developed this during our journey through life.

It is in this fundamental joy, in this happy knowledge that at bottom all is well with the world, that underneath the man-made sufferings God is with us and loves us, that we are sustained in imitating Christ gratefully and with open heart, and can receive what He said He had come to give us: life and joy.

> I came that they might have life and have it to the full.
>
> (John 10:10)
>
> All this I tell you that my joy may be yours and your joy may be complete.
>
> (John 15:11)

Finally, in a certain way, those psychiatrists you referred to are right, as the nuns were. Of course those psychiatrists have something quite different in mind when they say, "Be free and do as you like." But the Christian's goal *is* to become free—and not to be a slave of his emotions or sins—and to do as he likes (i.e., to develop a real liking for the moral good and to do it freely). But this happens only when the Christian's stony heart—the "heart" petrified by the overgrown "mind" of, e.g., the neurotic—has been replaced by a natural heart and a new spirit. With a new "heart" and spirit, the Christian is capable—if willing—of desiring to live according to God's statutes, and observe and carry out His ordinances. With the desire of the "heart" supporting the will, the Christian is free to do the good he likes. To help suffering people attain this goal is the task of the Christian psychiatrist.

Q. You keep talking about reason. But I have always been taught that we should live by faith, and that people who rely on reason are philosophers and not Christians. Are we not supposed to fear men's reason as part of the folly of the wise?

A. The Bible says, "I am not writing thus to shame you, but to bring you to reason" (1 Cor. 4:14 NEB). This is an example of the many times Paul speaks positively of reason. Reason, like all other aspects of our being and of our world, is perfected by faith, not negated by faith. "All things work together for the good of those who have been called according to his decree" (Rom. 8:28). Paul condemns the false worldly philosophies that do not acknowledge our total dependence on God, but he never gives up his reason. Why should God give us a faculty and then expect us not to use it?

Notice in Romans 1:20 that Paul lays it down as a basic part of his argument that all men can understand God's moral law through their reason alone, if they do not corrupt themselves by pride. Faith calls us to a total engagement of our faculties, to be as wise as serpents, which we sometimes must be to unsnarl the mysteries of our own psyches.

I trust you see again how unwise it is to think in terms of either/or. Reason *or* faith. Faith builds on reason; it takes over where reason leaves off. That is, if we are humble enough to admit that man cannot reason out everything for himself. And as the intellect builds on knowledge obtained from the senses, the mature man utilizes his senses *and* reason *and* intuitive mind *and* faith.

He does the same with the emotion of desire *and* will *and* hope. Together, his faith and hope, backed by the other modalities of knowing and striving, support love.

Q. You talk about my learning to exercise my own will, but the Scriptures teach, in the words of Jesus, "Not as I will, but as thou wilt" (Matt. 26:39 NEB). How can I be free to be me, and be God's servant at the same time?

A. We cannot will to do what God wills until our will is free and not encumbered by fear and a lack of faith and trust. We cannot will to surrender ourselves to God unless we possess ourselves in freedom. And unless God gives us the grace to do so. That is why it is so crucially important for the Christian psychiatrist to remove all psychological obstacles to his patient's freedom of will.

Q. Dr. Baars, this is not a question, just some comments and reflections. I have studied your writings

and those of Dr. Terruwe very carefully and recognized
without much difficulty that my troubles were those of
a lack of affirmation and a superimposed obsessive-
compulsive neurosis. I thought you may be interested
in hearing how I have applied your ideas to my personal
benefit, and also to my field of interest as a humanities
teacher.

The most troublesome part of my personality has
always been a deeply ingrained feeling of
worthlessness and guilt. I am convinced now that the
mortification of fear is the solution to this problem.
The constant feeling of anxiety, sudden surges of
inexplicable fear, the feeling of being off balance and
not quite rooted in one's own body, the awkward sense
of being perpetually displaced and threatened, the
restless and indeterminate strivings of a will that
knows not where to turn, since all avenues of action
lead to fear-inspiring ends—all those, which are
reminiscent of Thoreau's line, "I am a parcel of vain
strivings"—can only be dealt with by recognizing the
source from which they came originally (my mother,
long deceased), and experiencing the appropriate
anger, as often and as continuously as necessary to
restore equilibrium.

My mother was possessive, domineering, and an
expert "behavior manipulator" of her children. She
approved our existence only when we conformed to an
extension of herself. If not, she would create strong
feelings of fear and insecurity by threatening to leave
us. This scared us to death, for she would actually dress
as if she was getting ready to leave. She never was
satisfied with the way we felt, or what we did or said:
"You don't know what you want; you don't know what

you are doing; I don't know what's going to happen to you kids when I'm gone. When I die, who'll take care of you? What would you do without me to take care of you? You'll never learn to take care of yourself. Nobody ever cares about me. I wish I could die. You kids are killing me. How could you do that to your poor mother who loves you?"

Her disciplinary system was unpredictable. She changed rules all the time. She intimidated us with emotional displays. There were no certainties in my childhood emotional life, except we were sure to be made miserable every time we were happy. We were always told by her that whatever we *felt* was wrong, and that we should learn to *feel* like she did.

But to return to what is happening in "therapy." As I began to dare to feel anger at "Chairman Mother and her sayings," I noticed rumblings, little waves and ripples moving into my abdomen and upper chest. All my life, my upper chest and lower abdomen have been, literally, no-feeling zones, as well as certain parts of my face, the sources of my headaches—the result of retreat and paralyzed self in my childhood. This begins to explain the terrible deadness of my past life, and the inability to feel what others feel in poetry or times of sorrow and joy, the inability to let go. I couldn't let go because of the hypertrophy of fear, which I feared in turn; so every attempt to relax met with stubborn resistance. It was not until I learned the rational psychology of Aquinas-Terruwe-Baars that what I needed to let go was not the desire to relax, but anger. Now, whenever the old symptoms of fear make themselves felt, all I have to do is turn and face the monster with anger and a fierce will, and the relaxation of muscles sets in. Each time I do this, I feel myself change and grow, slowly but surely, in my feelings and emotions, with definite physical sensations accompanying the change.

I also understand now why my various excursions into Eastern techniques of relaxation were doomed to failure. They are all based on quietism. I wonder about the millions of people in our society, mostly young, who are in this same bind; they know there is something very wrong with them in terms of tension and anxiety, and they seek release where release is most obviously promised, in the stilling of the will altogether by negation of the personality. They see the Churches as *Ought* and *Hypocrisy,* experience that threat very vividly, see the tottering culture, and conclude that their inner problems can best be solved in the anomie of quietism. Drugs offer the same promise.

What we have as the most pervasive force in our declining culture is therefore a *psychological nihilism.* Value nihilism and revolutionary nihilism can gain so much credence among the young of the West because the psychological nihilism is already there to receive it, as a seed bed receives a seed. I see this more and more among my students and become more and more aware that it is espoused and encouraged by the liberal intelligentsia of academe, for it answers their purpose. It is often disguised as a form of existentialism. Faculties in the humanities tend to encourage despair, and punish all forms of optimism and religious commitment—even the theologians.

There are several books[48] which analyze, from different perspectives, our contemporary situation. Each sees the modern university as a place where grievous errors are taught as a matter of rote. In one book,[49] the author says our people are being devoured by a "fashionable existentialism" which drives us more and more to political suicide.

I think the roots lie deep in the psychological nihilism of the personality that emanates from so many focuses in our society. It is fashionable to feel despair and to be eaten up by *nausea à la Sartre,* to complain that there is no meaning, to deride all attempts to see the truth. Add that trend to the psyches of many a person already stunted by a Puritan culture, and you have the legitimizing of self-hate, self-hate given philosophical underpinnings and literary respectability.

In conclusion, I would like to comment on what is happening to my fantasy life since I began to try and live according to the principles described in your books. I have always been bothered by sinful thoughts and fantasies: pictures floating into my mind of what I would like to do, and enjoying those fantasies. As a child I was taught that such imagined deeds are as sinful as real deeds. Also that Jesus says that lusting in our hearts is just as evil as adultery.

I have discovered from your recommendations for obsessive-compulsive neurotics (in books and tapes) that when I do go ahead and be tolerant of my fantasies, the very fantasies that I used to try to stop, even when an apostate and away from the Church, that they began to change and develop in different directions or simply became boring after a while. At first, the luxuriating in the freedom of the imagination tended to run riot, but I can see already how this gets old and even silly. It is as if I am discovering "natural" reasons for abandoning sexual fantasies that before not even all my will power of moral "I must's" and "I should's" could succeed in destroying. In fact, I am quite sure that those sexual fantasies grew stronger over the years because of my trying so hard and sincerely to get rid of them. Sad to say, I never thought I was engaged in a neurotic process. Because parents, priests and sisters taught me that I must will away impure thoughts, etc., I thought I was doing what is normal and reasonable. And because I didn't succeed, I blamed myself, and considered myself weak and evil.

I want to thank you for having shown me the difference between rational guidance and neurotic repression of emotions, and for giving me courage to substitute "I may" for "I must." I am certain I will be healed, and that my love for God and His laws and commandments will grow from within me. How terribly sad it is that parents, teachers and religious used to think it necessary to *impose* moral behavior and love of God on children from without. It does not surprise me in the least that so many people have rebelled against excessive OUGHTism in their religion and upbringing, but have not found the answer either in total "freedom" and discarding of all moral laws and authority. Your ideas truly represent, in my opinion, the golden means which are psychologically and morally sound and responsible.

A. I am grateful for your sharing some of your experiences and your reflections on the "rational psychology of Aquinas-Terruwe-Baars." It is sad indeed that you had to suffer so unnecessarily, for it is evident that you are possessed of innate superior qualities which would have borne so much rich fruit for yourself and others, if you had been educated to be yourself, instead of trained to be like your mother. I hope you keep in touch with me, for I am sure that I can learn much from your profound insights.

Q. In Colossians 2:11, 12 (NEB), St. Paul says that by baptism I was "divested of my lower nature." I was baptized when I was a child, but I still feel the pull of lust very strongly, and it drives me to sin after sin. How do you explain this, and what can I do?

A. It is necessary to notice that Paul always follows such statements, as he does here in the remainder of this epistle, with statements that make explicit the need to actualize the gifts God has given. The gifts we receive in Baptism are often blocked and prevented from being actualized by some impediment, e.g., a prematurely instilled excessive OUGHT-consciousness. This must be healed first by the means I have described, before one's lower nature can cooperate with one's will and God's grace.

Remember that this is precisely the problem Paul was dealing with when he wrote to Jewish congregations who had been immersed in legalistic thinking—the problem of grace and law. Paul had to lead them to see that a whole new relationship to God's law had been revealed, through grace, which brings freedom of the spirit.

Notice also that many portions of Paul's epistles specifically admonish his missions congregations for falling into legalistic questions in a way that bespeaks scrupulosity and obsessive-compulsive behavior. That is why he keeps answering such questions by hammering away at the basic theme of freedom through grace, and a new, wholly new, relationship to the Law. If we treat Paul in a legalistic and overscrupulous manner, we are thoroughly missing his psychological and spiritual points. This would be a great pity, as Paul fully understood the need for proclaiming the new relationship to God inherent in Christ's grace, the fulfillment, not the alteration of the law, and the good news of the gospel which frees us to live in holiness by faith, not fear.

When you have begun to practice the recommendations of this book, you will learn experientially how this is so, and will turn to the Scriptures again with new eyes and new faith.

Q. When I was a child, almost everything I wanted to do was forbidden as soon as I showed an inclination in that direction. As a result, I have never been able to give up doing these things secretly, even though they make me feel guilty when I do them, and make me miserable most of the time. I feel I am on an endless treadmill. How do I get off?

A. The ultimate consequence of the oppressive—because excessive—*thou shalt not* mentality of parents and educators is always an obsession with the things they forbade and a compulsion to do those very same things.

When this is a treadmill of sexual "sins," and more often than not it is, the victim feels more guilty and evil than he would if he had landed on a nonsexual treadmill. He believes that sins against the sixth and ninth commandments are worse than those against the other eight, because they deal with sex.

Few people realize it is not the sexual drive per se and a weakness of the will that are responsible for compulsive sexual "sins." If parents, and other educators, were to make the same fuss about some of the other commandments, the child would land on a treadmill of lying or stealing, or something else.

In fact, one could set out and make of a child an obsessive-compulsive neurotic about virtually anything, provided the child has all the superior qualities I described earlier, and the parents and religious instructors instill—by their teachings, attitudes, behavior—the same fear or/and energy as regarding sex. Thus, if they wanted, they could create anything as ridiculous as a "chair neurosis," a "candy neurosis," a "doorknob neurosis," or what have you.

If there existed a religion that considered it a mortal sin to sit on a chair, to eat candy, to touch doorknobs, to take a shower, or whatever, all that would be necessary for adults to make their children develop a corresponding neurosis, is to pound from an early age on the dangers and terrible consequences of doing these particular things. In the gifted children fear or/and energy would then move them to be obedient and refrain from all such sinful actions. They would do so, with more or less near perfect success for a number of years, until later in life they would become increasingly obsessed with fantasies of sitting on a chair or eating candy, and finally end up being compelled to sit on a chair or eat the forbidden candy.

Those persons would then suffer the same intense feelings of guilt and shame, that are commonly experienced by the victims of "*over*exposure" to the sixth and ninth commandments. But they would have the advantage of finding it easier to comprehend and accept, once it is explained to them, that it is not their own evil nature that causes them to sin, but rather an outside cause. It also would be easier for them to become free by applying the principle of therapy: the mortification of the fear or/and energy of the chair, the candy, etc.

Q. I am always confused about guilt and guilt feelings. Are they the same?

A. When a person freely commits a crime or a sin, he *is* guilty of that crime or sin. Normally the awareness of his guilt is accompanied by a *feeling* of guilt. This feeling functions as a psychic motor to support his will to make restitution.

A psychopathic personality, on the other hand, does not have guilt feelings when he commits a crime. He may feel bad when he is caught, but not because he has done something wrong.

A neurotic often suffers from guilt feelings without having committed a crime or a sin. For example, a scrupulous person lives in constant fear that he has transgressed moral laws. This fear stimulates his guilt feelings, and vice versa.

Q. Not too long ago I read an article by a Dallas psychiatrist who stated, "Neither I nor my profession has the means to explain and predict the seemingly random acts of unprovoked violence that occasionally flash across front pages." If I remember correctly he cited violent TV programs and "dehumanization" as main factors. What is your opinion?

A. I do not know what exactly that psychiatrist meant by "dehumanization," but it could well refer to the effect on the personality of a child who did not grow up in the orbit of affirming parents and/or other significant others. When a child grows up feeling unloved, unwanted, worthless and unloveable he often considers and feels himself to be bad. As a result he not only will hate himself, but also those who denied him what he senses to be a fundamental human right. In some this hate may grow into a desire to take revenge and, if so, will lead to acts of violence against either the parents who have failed him, or any other authority figures.

In my opinion, this particular cause of unprovoked violence in our society is of greater, more fundamental, importance than the usual cited causes like war, TV violence, alcohol-induced violence in families, etc. The growing number of unstable families—because of divorce, working mothers, frequent geographical uprooting necessitated by job demands—and of unaffirmed parents contribute to a quantitative and qualitative increase in lack of emotional and intellectual affirmation. This is the primary cause for psychic weakness with fewer loving relationships, less respect for others, intensified polarization, more denial and rejection, etc. All this could well be summarized perhaps by the word "dehumanization."

Q. If it is true, as you say, that certain therapists and counselors employ ineffectual affirmation methods and techniques, how does a person in need of affirmation determine which therapists and institutes claiming to provide affirmation therapy actually do so in the true sense of the word? And how does one ascertain what affirmation books are reliable and authentic?

A. The answer to your questions is not a simple one. It is comparatively easy for people, especially when ill and in need of effective therapy, to be taken in by books and articles boasting of accomplishments and cures, and by solicitations containing favorable statements by well-known public figures. The same holds true for people in need of affirmation.

It would be well to keep in mind that the treatment of unaffirmed persons, particularly deprivation neurotics, was not generally known until recent times, and that therefore claims of large numbers of cures must be considered suspect. There simply has not been sufficient time to evaluate the results of this particular approach in a scientifically valid manner. There has been even less time for follow-up studies to differentiate between persons healed permanently and those who improved only as the result of living temporarily in a different environment, and had their original symptoms reappear after they had returned to their former milieu. Only Dr. Anna Terruwe in the Netherlands and I in the United States have treated deprivation neurotics and other unaffirmed persons for a sufficiently long period—approximately thirty and twenty years respectively—to have a reasonably accurate opinion of the results of our therapy.

A careful and critical evaluation of affirmation books, and for that matter, of all books on psychology, is always in order because of the fact that the field is noted for plagiarism. Whether copying the ideas of another author and passing off the same as one's original work occurs more often in psychology than in other fields of endeavor I do not know. The fact that it occurs is reason enough to proceed with caution in evaluating authors and therapists.

The introduction of such totally novel psychological terms as "affirmation," "deprivation neurosis" and "self-affirmation," and failure to indicate whether the author himself or someone else first coined these terms, is reason to suspect him of plagiarism. Not acknowledging the professional ideas of another person is a form of denial, the very opposite of affirmation. The introduction of the aforementioned terms in the Dutch and English-speaking psychiatric literature by Dr. Terruwe and myself is well documented and precisely dated. This fact will facilitate any investigation of authors of affirmation books.

An author focusing primarily or solely on emotional affirmation while ignoring or slighting the role of intellectual affirmation is likely to have less than adequate knowledge of the subject. To describe the latter as "encouragement to develop one's intellectual capacities, to take more schooling and take delight in one's intellect," betrays great ignorance on the part of the writer. It might even indicate the possibility of plagiarism, and a poor job at that.

A person who writes in glowing terms about affirmation while only casually referring to the evil of self-affirmation either has not given the subject deep thought, or is possibly blind to that quality in himself—many of us are poor self-evaluators—and is trying to affirm himself by taking credit for ideas that are not his own. As I explained in *Born Only Once*, one form of self-affirmation consists of trying to become famous by any means, or of associating with famous persons.

A statement in the preface of a book that the author does "not have the intention of repeating what he has acknowledged elsewhere" will make any reader wonder what he has to hide, and why. Even if the writer has done what he says he did, how is the reader to know which person had the original ideas used by the author in his book? In my opinion, the reader owes it to himself, and perhaps also to those entrusted to his care, to demand that the author give the proper acknowledgments and make it clear whether he or someone else deserves the credit for originality.

If a writer seems to be a name-dropper and quotes persons of note who are unlikely to be personally acquainted with his work, as if they support it, one would be advised to check this out with them. One should ask them whether they were quoted correctly, or ever had the intention to speak in support of the author, and if so, whether they still hold the same opinion. It could well be that their opinion has changed, or that their statement was never supposed to express approval or support of that author in the first place. Name-dropping should be particularly suspect if the names are of persons who are not easy to contact, for instance, because of their high position in the Church or their place of residence in a foreign country.

Lastly, in 1976 Dr. Terruwe and I found it necessary to retain an attorney to put a certain author on notice that unless "any reference to the thoughts, words and ideas of Drs. Terruwe and Baars be properly cited and attributed in his intended publication—a book on affirmation—any such plagiarism may result in legal action for damages." Suffice it to say that the author in question decided to ignore this notice. When someone claims to be an affirmer, yet does not practice what he preaches, he is not an affirmer of others.

Q. In discussions about the seeming increase of violence in our society and world many persons seem to assume as a fact that human beings have an inborn aggressive drive. Do you agree with this notion?

A. I certainly do not. If one agrees with Webster's definition of "aggression" as an "attack without provocation," then it is certain that man does not have an inherited, biological and fixed instinct or drive to be aggressive. Contrary to what many authors claim in order to justify violence as if it were a natural catastrophe, although man has the capacity to attack others without provocation he is not genetically fated to do so.

In fact, the very opposite is true. Man has a fundamental, natural tendency to love and respect the well-being and integrity of his fellow-men. It is possible that some persons mistake man's innate drive to self-realization for an aggressive drive. However, this drive aims at the development of his innate potentialities, talents, character, etc., and may cause him to be assertive when obstacles to the fulfillment of this drive are placed in his way. His capacity to be assertive thus serves his innate drive for self-realization—and for that matter also his other innate drive, that of procreation. Assertiveness must be clearly distinguished from aggressiveness if we are to understand the nature of man. "Assertive," again according to Webster, means: "(1) characterized by, or disposed to affirm, to declare with assurance, to state positively; (2) to maintain or defend, e.g., one's rights or prerogatives."

Q. Is there a difference between "impulsive" and "compulsive"?

A. Indeed there is, and a very important one at that. These two words are sometimes used interchangeably and thus cause confusion. "Impulse" is a sudden, involuntary inclination or feeling which prompts the person to action. If he does act without reflecting on the possible consequences, like a child does or a psychopathic personality, he acts *impulsively*, or on impulse! Impulsiveness characterizes the child, the immature adult, and the psychopath.

"Compulsion," on the other hand, describes the irresistible need to perform certain acts, even though the person does not will to do them, either because they are senseless, useless or contrary to his moral convictions. These compulsive acts are typical of the obsessive-compulsive neurotic who is driven to perform those acts in order to achieve some temporary and transient respite of his chronic anxiety and tension.

Some of these persons are compelled to painstakingly clean everything they have touched over and over again, usually for fear that others may be harmed by dirt or germs. Others compulsively wash their hands and forearms with soap twenty or thirty times a day, even when they know that it makes no sense and creates needless disturbance in the home for spouse and children. Like compulsive masturbation, these actions represent the ultimate breakdown of the chronic repressive process and are proof of the fact that the person's will has been eliminated from dealing with the repressed emotions. That person is incapable of utilizing his free will in the area of repression, while being free in other areas, e.g., in matters of honesty. In other words, though compelled to masturbate, he is not compelled in the least to rob a bank.

In this connection it is well to discuss briefly another term akin to compulsion, namely "perfectionism." The intense striving to do things as perfectly as possible is seen most frequently in unaffirmed people who want to gain the acceptance, praise and love of others. It is learned in childhood, especially when the inadequately affirming parents are also difficult to please and constantly demand more of the child. Unlike the behavior of the obsessive-compulsive neurotic, that of the perfectionist is not irrational or senseless, but rather appropriate even though carried to an extreme. The greater the person's need for love and acceptance the more intense the need to do things perfectly.

Because an obsessive-compulsive neurosis can coexist with a deprivation neurosis in one and the same person, it follows that compulsiveness and perfectionism can be seen together also. This, of course, explains why even professionals may use these two terms as being synonymous and confuse the patient. But recognition of the syndrome of nonaffirmation can bring the clarity required for diagnostic and therapeutic purposes.

Q. Are "selfishness" and "self-centeredness" the same?

A. I am glad you asked me that question. I see so many patients in my practice who consider themselves selfish, while all they are is self-centered or egocentric. Virtually every person, even the most unselfish and "other-centered" one, will focus his attention on himself, when, for example, he becomes sick or disabled by an accident. By doing so he will move to seek the necessary help or treatment. His self-centeredness is a necessary condition for self-preservation. It will be present only as long as he is in need of help or treatment. Once this has been given, his self-centeredness will be replaced, if he is normally so disposed, by his usual concern and interest in others. Of course, when his suffering is chronic, like it is in neurotic conditions, the person is, of necessity, self-centered all of the time, or most of the time, even when of an unselfish and generous bent.

Selfishness, or egotism on the other hand, is something entirely different. The selfish person cares only for himself. He is self-seeking, and not in the sense that he is searching for his own identity! His own interests come first, even at the expense of the welfare of others. This extreme degree of selfishness is typical of the psychopathic personality. In less severe form, selfishness is characteristic of all human beings, since it is the primary consequence of original sin. A selfish person is always self-centered, but the reverse is not necessarily true. The self-centered neurotic who is also generous and unselfish in his suffering makes quite a different impression on all of us than the not-sick person who is decidedly selfish (e.g., self-affirming persons).

Q. People often say that I always feel sorry for myself and that I should stop doing that. How do I get rid of my self-pity?

A. I don't think it wrong to feel sorry for yourself. If it were, it would also be wrong to feel sorry for others who are in trouble or miserable. Yet, nobody every reproaches a person for feeling sorry for others. The explanation for this is that we usually do something for the persons who are miserable and stir our pity; we give them alms or help them in some other ways that will make life more pleasant for them.

But this is not always the case when we feel sorry for ourselves. Either because we do not know what to do, or lack the courage to get ourselves out of the mess we are in, we feel sorry for ourselves without trying to change the situation. It is that lack of action which people reproach us for. They criticize our self-pity because it is not followed by activities aimed at alleviating our own misery. Perhaps we prefer to wait until others start to feel sorry for us, too. However, we cannot always count on that and should not compound that miscalculation by remaining stuck passively in our self-pity. The least we can do is to ask somebody else to help us, if we are unable to free ourselves from our pitiful situation.

Q. Dr. Baars, some time ago you said, I believe, that God does not punish us with hell. If so, do you mean by this that there is no hell, or that God never punishes?

A. I do indeed believe that there is a hell. In fact, for me its existence is another proof of God's infinite love for us. God loves us so much that He wants us to have everything we freely will to have. Having created man with a free will, and being a perfectly just God who created us for happiness, He wants to give us always our just due. If we will to be united with Him in love our just due is to be with Him in heaven. If we will to have nothing to do with Him, if we freely reject Him, then our just due is to be separated from Him. Therefore, in order to give us what we freely will to have, God had to create a "place" where He is not. That "place" we know as hell.

Let me further illustrate the extent and depth of the meaning of God's justice. If I were to reject God freely, He would be unjust to me if He would refuse to let me go to hell, and instead insist on admitting me to heaven. The nature of free will demands that I *must* be given what is owed me by virtue of my free choice. In this hypothetical case, God "must" let me go to hell.

Whether my going to hell is properly called punishment, is another matter. I don't think I have to go into this now.

Q. I grew up a Catholic, and in those days, long since gone by, I often heard talk about "concupiscence." I don't know exactly what the word means, but I got the impression it was something bad within us, something we should rid ourselves of. Can you explain this? Also, could you say something more about "mortification"? I got the impression when you mentioned this topic before that you are critical of it. Yet, you obviously are against the unbridled indulgence of feelings and emotions. I am sorry if I have missed the point and am asking you to repeat yourself.

A. I did not use the word "concupiscence" in this book for the very reason you mentioned; it is a misleading word that too often conveys a pejorative meaning it does not actually have.

Not too long ago a dogmatic theologian of renown criticized the ideas I had presented at a national congress of religious, and "felt compelled in conscience" to exclude my address from the congress's printed symposium. One of his several criticisms of my talk read: "Christ did not have a fallen human nature; He had no concupiscence," and also: "Dr. Baars is mistaken if he thinks Adam and Eve had concupiscence before the Fall, which is doctrinally impossible." Obviously, according to this critic, a proponent of the voluntaristic philosophy I mentioned before, concupiscence does not belong to human nature in its perfect state.

Yet "Aquinas defines concupiscence as the appetite for pleasure. . . . Pleasure, even sensible bodily pleasure, is not evil of itself. As the author of nature, God has placed pleasure in the exercise of certain natural operations, and especially those which pertain to the conservation of the individual and of the species."[50]

Judging by a dictionary's definition, concupiscence is: (1) sensual appetite; lust, (2) eager or illicit desire," in our daily language the voluntaristic (Ignatius, Suarez) meaning of the word has won out over the intellectualistic one (Thomas Aquinas). Concupiscence, a good in itself, has become synonymous with "disordered concupiscence." For this very reason I never use the word. As you already know I prefer "pleasure appetite" or "humane emotions."

"Mortification" is another troublesome term. According to the dictionary it means "the practice of asceticism by penetential discipline to overcome desire for sin and to strengthen the will."

You are already aware that I consider it a poor choice of words from a psychological point of view, because the Latin word, *mortificare*, means "to kill, to destroy." Nevertheless, I am in full agreement with the teaching that ascetical (from the Greek verb, *askētik(ós)*, meaning "to exercise" or "work hard") practices or exercises are necessary to foster the integration between emotions and reason and will. In fact, I advocate an even wider application of these exercises. The Church has always stressed the mortification of the emotions of the pleasure appetite more so than those of the utility appetite. However, since *both* appetites have suffered in their original relationship to reason and will as the result of Original Sin, it follows that *both* need to be mortified, or tempered, equally. Yet, as I have explained, the utilitarian emotions of fear and energy have been frequently the subject of stimulation, rather than mortification, in the expectation that this would promote virtuous living. My opinion of this you already know.

Our understanding of the role of irrational fear and excessive energy in the development of the obsessive-compulsive neuroses explains the need for the mortification of these utilitarian emotions. Moreover, it can be said that the mortification of these emotions, in a certain sense, is of a higher order than the asceticism of the emotions of the pleasure appetite.

Most of us tend to do what the obsessive-compulsive neurotic does in the extreme, namely, to attain our sanctification by our own energetic efforts and fearful attitudes. For some reason we prefer this, impossible as it is, to putting all our trust in God and surrendering ourselves to Him in faith. Yet, this is precisely what the Christian must do to such a degree that he cannot but perform good works willingly and gladly.

For the obsessive-compulsive neurotic that is the hardest thing to learn, much harder than the mortification of the emotions of the pleasure appetite, even though he usually is already an expert at this. Yet, he too, when assisted by an understanding and compassionate therapist can learn to live the Little Way of St. Teresa of Lisieux, the way of faith and surrender.

It is my sincerest wish that all this will eventually also be understood by voluntaristic theologians, who, to quote the aforementioned critic, object to the idea that "repression via Catholic teaching is the basis of emotionally *misfit* (his term, not mine!) Catholics."

Q. Do you meet with much opposition to the ideas you have presented in this book?

A. From time to time these ideas have been attacked and even condemned by officials in the Catholic Church. These critics have been few in number, but because of the high position of some, they had great impact. My colleague, Dr. Anna Terruwe, suffered for fifteen years from the condemnation of her ideas and work by the Holy Office in Rome. This, in spite of the fact that all the Dutch bishops and their own moral theologians, after conducting a full-scale investigation of certain allegations—made by certain proponents of the voluntaristic philosophy—and a hearing of Dr. Terruwe personally, had concluded that she was *orthodox in doctrina et prudens in praxi* ("orthodox in her teachings and prudent in their clinical applications").

Finally, one year after she wrote, for private use, a seventy-five-page exposé[51] of all that had transpired, the Holy Office in 1965 broke a decade of silence and refusal to respond to Dr. Terruwe's communications, and publicly expressed its regrets, declared "her work to be founded on sound and correct principles and of great value to all," and offered to make reparation for the harm done to her good name and professional reputation. Not long thereafter His Holiness Pope Paul VI twice requested a private consultation with my colleague. On one of these occasions he called her work and ideas—many of which are contained in the pages of this book—"*a gift to the Church.*"

Because of the widespread publicity that ensued in the Netherlands and abroad, her thoughts and pioneering work are now generally known and respected by professionals and nonprofessionals alike in much of western Europe. They received special recognition from an eminent Dutch psychiatrist in a small book, entitled, *The Significance of the Work of Dr. A.A.A. Terruwe for Psychiatry.*[52]

Postscript

"The truth that we owe to man is, first and foremost, a truth about man.

"Perhaps one of the most obvious weaknesses of present-day civilization lies in an inadequate view of man.

"Without doubt, our age is the one in which man has been most written and spoken of, the age of the forms of humanism and the age of anthropocentrism. Nevertheless it is paradoxically also the age of man's deepest anxiety about his identity and his destiny, the age of man's abasement to previously unsuspected levels, the age of human values trampled on as never before.

"How is this paradox explained?

"We can say that it is the inexorable paradox of atheistic humanism. It is the drama of man being deprived of an essential dimension of his being, namely his search for the infinite, and thus faced with having his being reduced in the worst way.

"Thanks to the Gospel . . . the truth about man . . . is found in an anthropology . . . whose primordial affirmation is that man is God's image."

I shall be deeply grateful to God if the ideas presented in this book contribute in some way to "a truth about man" as spoken of by Pope John Paul II in his first major address of his papacy to the 300 Latin American cardinals, bishops, priests and religious at Puebla, Mexico, in January, 1979.

His words underscore the meaning and spirit of what I consider my task and that of every Christian psychiatrist: to assist the Church and all Christians in knowing more about man as the image of God, to lessen his anxieties, to save him from his own abasement, and to bring order and strength to his psychic life for optimal receptivity to God's healing grace.

NOTA BENE

Readers of this book wanting to obtain a better understanding of themselves in the light of what the author has presented in these pages, and perhaps wanting to seek assistance in reaching a greater degree of psychic wholeness, are invited to send for any of the following:

1. List of available self-help cassettes, books, articles and monographs.

2. Information about arrangements for lectures, seminars, conferences, retreats, "workshops," by the author.

3. Suggestions for obtaining the author's professional consultation and help in recognizing and treating their

personal emotional-spiritual problems.

In addition, the author welcomes readers' comments, questions or discussion regarding the subject matter presented in this book. He also invites contact with interested professionals, persons in the healing ministry and departments of psychology and psychiatry in this country and abroad for the purposes of:

1. referring persons in need of counseling and healing.
2. advising students wanting to broaden their knowledge of rational and faculty psychology.
3. disseminating and stimulating interdisciplinary knowledge and study of "a truth about man."

All inquiries and correspondence, accompanied with a self-addressed, stamped, long envelope, should be addressed to:

C.W. Baars, M.D.
326 Highview Drive
San Antonio, Texas 78228

NOTES

[1]Mary R. Joyce, *The Impotent Playboy*, in preparation.
[2]"The New Narcissism," *Newsweek*, Jan. 30, 1978, p. 70.
[3]Mary R. Joyce and Robert E. Joyce, Ph.D., *New Dynamics in Sexual Love*, (St. John's University Press, Collegeville, Minn., 1970).
[4]A.A.A. Terruwe, M.D., *Psychopathic Personality and Neurosis*, and *The Neurosis in the Light of Rational Psychology*, transl. by Conrad W. Baars, M.D. (P.J. Kenedy & Sons, New York, 1958 and 1960 respect., both out of print).
A.A.A. Terruwe, M.D. and Conrad W. Baars, M.D., *Loving and Curing the Neurotic* (Arlington House, New Rochelle, NY, 1972, out of print).
Conrad W. Baars, M.D. and A.A.A. Terruwe, M.D., *Healing the Unaffirmed*, (Alba House, Staten Island, NY, 1976).
Conrad W. Baars, M.D. and A.A.A. Terruwe, M.D., *Healing for Neurotics*, (Alba House, Staten Island, NY, in prep.).
[5]by Carl Goldberg, M.D. in *Psychiatric Annals*, 7:11, Nov. 1977.
[6]from *The Spiritual Exercises of St. Ignatius* (The Newman Press, Westminster, Md., 1957).
[7]Max Weber, *The Protestant Ethic and The Spirit of Capitalism* (Chas. Scribner's Sons, NY, 1958) pp. 114 and 166.
[8]*Passio nata est obedire rationi.*
[9]The voluntaristic philosophy dates back to the *agere contra* (to act against) doctrine of St. Ignatius and Francisco Suarez, S.J.
[10]see also Conrad W. Baars, M.D., *A Priest for All Seasons—Masculine and Celibate*, and *Crisis in the Priesthood*, (Franciscan Herald Press, Chicago, IL, 1972).
[11]see Josef Pieper, *Guide to Thomas Aquinas*, (Pantheon Books, 1962).
[12]W.J.A.J. Duynstee, C.SS.R., LL.D., *De Verdringingstheorie beoordeeld van thomistisch standpunt*, 1935.
[13]C.W. van Boekel, "Catharsis," *Een filologische reconstructie van de psychologie van Aristoteles omtrent het gevoelsleven*, (De Fontein, Utrecht, 1957).
Other references regarding Aquinas' original views of man's emotional life:
J.P. van Boxtel, "Moraal en Affectiviteit," in *De Menselyke Persoon in de Christelyke Moraal*, 1958.
J.P. van Boxtel, "Moraal en Gevoelsleven volgens Thomas van Aquino," in *Tydschrift voor Philosophie*, June 1959.
Stephanus Pfürtner, O.P., *Triebleben und Sittliche Vollendung—Eine Moralpsychologische Untersuchung nach Thomas von Aquin*, (Universitätsverlag, Freiburg, Schweiz, 1958).

[14]F. Veldman, *Life Welcomed and Affirmed*, (Academie voor Haptonomie en Kinesionomie, Nymegen, Netherlands, 1976).

[15]Dr. Frederick Boyer, *Birth Without Violence*, (A.A. Knopf, NY 1975).

[16]i.e., sinful in itself, as opposed to "subjective," meaning "sinful for that particular person in his particular circumstances.

[17]Several deprivation neurotics have told me that they feel guilty because of the Prayer of St. Francis: "Where there is hatred, let me sow love," (but they are incapable of doing this), and also, "Grant that I may not so much seek to be loved as to love," (yet they need to seek and find love).

[18]*Diagnostic and Statistical Manual of Mental Disorders*, second ed., (American Psychiatric Association, 1968).

[19]*The Neurosis in the Light of Rational Psychology* and *Loving and Curing the Neurotic*.

[20]see my comment on May's discussion of self-affirmation in Conrad W. Baars, M.D., *Born Only Once*, (Franciscan Herald Press, Chicago, IL, 1975).

[21]see also *Psychopathic Personality and Neurosis*, pp. 21-77.

[22]Conrad W. Baars, M.D., *The Homosexual's Search for Happiness*, (Franciscan Herald Press, Chicago, IL 1976).

[23]I am grateful to Barbara Shlemon, R.N., author of *Healing Prayer*, for sharing this information with me.

[24]For information on how to obtain these self-help tapes please consult the postscript of this book.

[25]Gal. 5:22 and 1 Cor. 12:4-11, respectively.

[26]see for example, *Loving and Curing the Neurotic*, pp. 210-211, and *Healing the Unaffirmed*, pp. 76-87.

[27]see Chapter 8, p. 213

[28]*The American College Dictionary*, (Random House, 1953).

[29]Summa Theologica, II, II, 153, 3.

[30]Professionals interested in learning more about the spiritual aspects of healing can receive information from at least two sources: Association of Christian Therapists, 2213 Cherry Street, Toledo, OH 43608.

International Order of St. Luke the Physician, Editorial Office, 1787 Goodrich Ave., St. Paul, Minn. 55105; *Sharing* magazine, St. Luke's Press, 61 Broad Street, Elizabeth, NJ 07201.

Recommended basic reading on spiritual healing:

Francis MacNutt, O.P., *Healing*, (Ave Maria Press, Notre Dame, Ind., 1974).

Francis MacNutt, O.P., *The Power to Heal*, (Ave Maria Press, 1977).

Agnes Sanford, *The Healing Light*, (Logos International, Plainfield, NJ 1972).

[31]For information on how to obtain my self-help tapes on Forgiveness and Inner Healing, please consult the postscript at the end of this book.

[32]Steve Clark, *Emotions in the Christian Life*, 6 tape cassettes, Foundations of Christian Living Series, (The Word of God, Ann Arbor, Mich.).

[33]David H. Barlow, Ph.D., Gene G. Abel, M.D., and Edward B. Blanchard, "Gender Identity Change in a Transsexual: An Exorcism," *Archives of Sexual Behavior*, Vol. 6, No. 5, 1977.

[34]John J. Schwab, M.D., "Psychiatry's Identity Crisis," *Psychiatric Opinion*, April 1978; "Psychiatry Runs Into an Identity Crisis, *U.S. News and World Report*, Oct. 9, 1978.

[35]*Clinical Psychiatry News*, June 1978.

[36]*Psychiatric News*, Oct. 20, 1978.

[37]see Alexander Solzhenitsyn, *A World Split Apart*, address given at the Harvard commencement exercises, June 8, 1978.

[38]*Hypothetical Dilemmas for Use in Moral Discussion*, Moral Education and Research Foundation of Harvard.

[39]It seems difficult to believe that in some Catholic dioceses all priests were ordered by their Ordinaries to attend the entire "workshop in spiritual growth," developed by Rev. V. Dwyer, OCSO, designed by Fathers Weber and Kilgallon of ACTA Foundation, and directed by the National Catholic Reporter Publishing Co. Reportedly, these priests also had to submit to psychological testing before and after the 18 sessions workshop by Father Dwyer's trained staff, and all behavior responses (e.g., dropping out) were kept on file. The facilitator's handbook (Genesis II—bridges the gap between the old and the new. Copyright Intermedia Foundation, 1975) contains a 2 page bibliography listing among others Rollo May, Margaret Mead, Abraham Maslow, Eric Fromm, Eugene Kennedy, Marc Oraison, Hans Kung, Gabriel Moran, John McKensie.

[40]A casuist is one who studies and resolves cases of conscience or conduct.

[41]*The Neurosis in the Light of Rational Psychology*.

[42]"We ourselves have seen many unaffirmed persons . . . among our alcoholic patients, and we have been struck repeatedly by the reports of authors who, in attempting to describe an alcoholic personality, almost always mention the main symptoms of the deprivation neurotic. To quote, for example, from a recent psychiatric study which describes a *characteristic life style, rather than specific personality traits* of the alcoholic: 'A deeply felt sense of inadequacy is invariably present. . . . The earliest memories center on damage or abandonment, and the reaction of helplessness. . . . A distinctive hypersensitivity is present,

especially noticeable in personal relationships and in attitudes about talent, creativity, and success. Achievement is frequently discounted and is not experienced as success or as the fulfillment of genuine ambition. . . .'

"And from a widely circulated book by a recovered alcoholic and respected member of A.A. we quote: 'Too dependent throughout his life on some person . . . feels insecure, incompetent, and childlike . . . essentially a lonely class of people . . . anxious, fearful and tense in the real world . . . the central desire of his whole nature is that of being caressed by his mother . . . the source of his craving for attention is often a lack of self-confidence . . . failure to accept and love himself.'

"The relatively few remaining personality features are typical of the repressive neurotics, and another few of the psychopathic personality disorders. . . . The latter have little or no need to seek relief in alcohol, as they suffer very little tension or anxiety. . . .'

"The insight based on this classification explains . . . why alcoholics require specific psychiatric treatment if they are to enjoy lasting quality sobriety. The unaffirmed alcoholic needs in addition to active A.A. membership, one kind of psychotherapy; the repressive neurotic alcoholic another; some a combination of the two. . . .'

"Interestingly, the distrust if not complete rejection by many A.A. members of psychoanalytic therapy for alcoholics finds its justification in our particular aristotelian-thomistic interpretation of emotional illnesses. We believe that psychoanalysis is indicated only in hysterical neurotics, who constitute a very small percentage of the repressive neurotics, and, of course, an even smaller percentage of all neurotics. . . . It follows that only a very small number of alcoholics can be expected to benefit from this particular type of psychiatric treatment." (from "The Alcoholic Priest," by Conrad W. Baars, M.D., *The Priest*, Vol. 27, No. 6, June 1971)

[43]The title of Dr. Abraham Low's textbook. Dr. Low was the founder of Recovery, Inc.

[44]*Weekend Overview–A support document for the Worldwide Marriage Encounter–Weekend Outline*, 1978.

[45]from a chapter by Mary S. Calderone, M.D. in *The New Sex Education*, Herbert A. Otto, (ed.), Follett, Chicago, 1978. Dr. Calderone is the president of SIECUS (Sex Information and Education Council of the United States), editor of *Abortion in the United States*, and *Manual of Family Planning and Contraceptive Practice;* and past Medical Director of the Planned Parenthood Federation of America.

[46]Mary R. Joyce, *How Can a Man and Woman be Friends?* (The Liturgical Press, Collegeville, Minn. 1977).

[47]see *Healing the Unaffirmed*, pp. 185-9.

[48]Christopher Derrick, *Escape from Scepticism*, Thomas Aquinas College.

John Senior, *The Death of Christian Culture*, (Arlington House, 1978).

Thomas Molnar, *On Christian Humanism: A Critique of the Ideology of the Secular City* (Franciscan Herald Press, Chicago, 1978).

Jacques Ellul, *Betrayal of the West*, (Seabury Press, NY, 1978).

[49]Saul Bellow, *To Jerusalem & Back*, (The Viking Press, NY, 1977).

[50]Antonio Royo, O.P. and Jordan Aumann, O.P., *The Theology of Christian Perfection* (The Priory Press, Dubuque, Iowa, 1962) p. 264.

[51]A.A.A. Terruwe, M.D., *Opening van Zaken, In Usum Privatum*, (Nymegen, 1964).

[52]Prof. Dr. J.J.G. Prick, *De Betekenis van het Werk van Dr. A.A.A. Terruwe voor de Psychiatrie*, (De Tydstroom, 1973).

INDEX